Student Survival Guide

From Here to Eternity

Edited by
Deborah Glover
and
Phillip Hufton

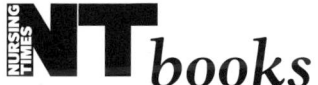

First published 1999 by Nursing Times Books
Emap Healthcare Ltd, part of Emap Business Communications
Greater London House
Hampstead Road
London NW1 7EJ

Text © 1999 Emap Healthcare Ltd

Typeset & Glossary graphics drawn by Joanna Chalmers, Bertiesoft Ltd, Oxted, Surrey
Cover design: Senate Design Ltd, London
Cover images courtesy of The Moviestore Collection Ltd, London

Printed and bound in Great Britain by Thanet Press Ltd, Margate, Kent

All rights reserved. No reproduction, copy or transmission of this publication may be made without written permission. No paragraph of this publication may be reproduced, copied or transmitted save with the written permission of the publisher or in accordance with the provisions of the Copyright, Designs and Patents Act 1988 or under the terms of any licence permitting limited copying issued by the Copyright Licensing Agency, 90 Tottenham Court Road, London W1P 0LP.

Any person who does any unauthorised act in relation to this publication may be liable to criminal prosecution and civil claims for damages.

British Library cataloguing in Publication Data
A catalogue record for this book is available from the British Library.

ISBN: 1 902499 22 0

Foreword

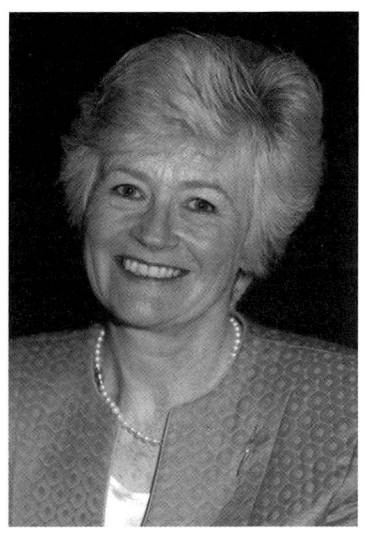

Dame Yvonne Moores,

Chief Nursing Officer/ Director of Nursing

This book is aimed at the many women and men who have chosen nursing or midwifery for their future career. You are about to embark on an exciting journey of learning and self-discovery, of dedication and commitment.

My own career started 40 years ago, and has continued through different governments, advances in medical science and technology, and many changes in the philosophies and theories which drive nursing.

For example, the word 'vocation' became unfashionable for a while – it was felt to characterise an unassertive nursing world led by soft and woolly 'do-gooders'. It had religious connotations, meaning a 'calling'. It lacked professional credibility in the hard-edged world of a male dominated medical culture. Yet every nurse will recall the individual moment when he or she first made a real, meaningful connection with a patient or client. The first smile, after many months of working with a severely learning disabled client. The first time you feel confident enough to handle difficult questions from a patient with terminal cancer. The first time you witness the birth of a baby. The first time you draw up an injection without feeling utterly uncoordinated and incompetent. The first time an elderly confused patient greets you with warmth and recognition.

These personal achievements and relationships are the essence of the nursing 'vocation'. But behind them lies the substantial foundation of theory – an understanding of anatomy and physiology, the recognition of the patient's psychological state, the appreciation of pharmacology and biosciences, and the knowledge of how society and communities work. Beyond this basic core of knowledge lies the ability to practise, manage, research and teach in the complex environment of the modern day health service. It is this core knowledge that secures the place of nursing, midwifery and health visiting as the backbone of the NHS, and so many other care sectors.

Nursing is an art, and a science. Nursing is rational, yet allows for emotion. And – most importantly – nurses make a difference.

As you start out on your journey, and as I retire after mine, I truly hope that you will share with me the happiness, friendship and self-fulfilment that my own nursing career has brought to me.

Good luck!

Yvonne Moores

August 1999

Contents

Foreword   iii
Dame Yvonne Moores, Chief Nursing Officer/Director of Nursing

Meet the contributors   viii

Introduction   xii
Deborah Glover and Phillip Hufton

1. The Getting of Wisdom – a light-hearted introduction to student life   1
   Mark Radcliffe

2. The Way We Were – the history of nursing   14
   Marsh Gelbart
   Chaos, class and contradictions p.14, From ritual to research p.17, Poverty pay p.18, Appalling accommodation p.19, Status and sciatica p.20

3. Being There – preparation for theory and practice   22
   Erica Forth
   Be afraid, very afraid! p.22, Great expectations (not) p.23, Realistic expectations p.25

4. The Defiant Ones – the students' union explained   27
   Andrew Garland
   Purpose of the students' union p.28, The university system p.28, The students' union and the National Union of Students p.29, Students' union services p.29, Structure of a union p.30, Getting involved p.30, Adapting services to nursing students p.32

Student survival guide

5 The Empire Strikes Back – an explanation of the NHS   35
   Eileen Walsh
   The early days p.35, Moving into the 20th century p.36, Creating the NHS p.37, Organisational changes in the NHS p.38, The NHS in England p.40, Variations on the NHS across the UK p.44, Feeding the beast: funding the NHS p.46, What lies ahead? p.47

6 The Matrix – glossary of terms/anatomical positions   48
   Phillip Hufton
   Medical terminology p.48, Roots p.49, Suffixes p.52, Anatomical position p.53, Abbreviations p.56

7 Other People's Money – managing your finances   59
   Zosia Kmietowicz
   What is a bursary? p.59, How much is a bursary? p.59, Extra financial assistance p.61, Boosting your bursary p.63, Budgeting p.63, How to survive – basic dos and don'ts when living on a low income p.64, Making your money go further p.65, Useful contacts p.66

8 Payback – where to find help and support   69
   Andrew Garland
   Starting out p.69, Advice available p.70, Who can help? p.71, Who should help? p.71, What can be improved? p.72, Students' union welfare p.73, Counselling p.74, Health promotion p.74, Money p.75, Finding out more p.76, Useful website addresses p.76

9 The Net – information technology in healthcare   78
   Ken Campbell
   Types of software p.79, Sources of software p.82, The Internet and the World Wide Web p.84, Citing electronic resources in academic writing p.85

10 The Pure Hell of St Trinian's – academic hints and tips   87
   Janet Hesketh
   Lectures p.88, Discussions, tutorials and seminars p.90,

Contents

Writing essays and assignments p.93, Preparing for examinations p.97, Presentations p.100

11 Up Close and Personal – personal experiences of training   102
Lee Bickley, Yvonne Bossons, Jessica Cudmore and Paul Smith Roberts

12 Alien Nation – the other contributors to healthcare   109
Jill Newman

Medical staff p.110, Professions allied to medicine p.112, Professional and technical staff p.115, Administrative and clerical staff p.115, Estate management and ancillary services p.116, External agencies p.118

13 Do the Right Thing – accountability, professionalism and whistleblowing   119
Deborah Glover and Dr Geoffrey Hunt

Accountability to the public p.121, Accountability to the employer p.122, Accountability to the patient p.124, Accountability to the profession p.129, Whistleblowing p.131

14 Desperately Seeking Susan – useful contacts   136
Martin Vousden

15 Reality Bites – what to expect once you qualify   156
Tony Makepeace

Registration p.156, Which job? p.157, The application form p.158, The interview p.159, Preceptorship and 'reality shock' p.160, Project 2000 p.162, Education p.163, Money p.163

16 Carry on Nurse – nursing howlers   168
Phillip Hufton

Meet the contributors

Ken Campbell

Ken Campbell has over 15 years' experience as a medical laboratory scientific officer, having obtained Fellowship of the Institute of Biomedical Sciences in 1984. He is currently employed as information officer for the Leukaemia Research Fund. He is a member of the British Society for Haematology, the European Haematology Association and the Society for the Internet in Medicine. He is currently involved in the discussion groups relating to the proposed Electronic Library for Health. He has written a number of articles for *Nursing Times* on leukaemia and related topics.

Erica Forth

Erica Forth is an E-grade staff nurse at Salford Hospital.

Andrew Garland

Having been encouraged by its move into higher education, Andrew began his nurse training in April 1996 at the age of 29. He represents the interests of student nurses at the students' union, University of Wales, Bangor. He has every intention of remaining actively involved in the Association of Nursing Students until he qualifies in April 2000. After qualifying he hopes to be in a position to encourage students to take up active roles within both the RCN and students' unions.

Marsh Gelbart

Marsh qualified in Sheffield in 1981 and has worked as a nurse in Britain and abroad. He worked at the London Lighthouse in HIV/AIDS as a primary nurse for five years before working as a health adviser at the John Hunter Clinic, HIV/GUM Directorate at the Chelsea and Westminster Trust, London. He is currently a temporary lecturer at the Wolfson School of Health Studies, Thames Valley University, and writes on health affairs as a freelancer.

Meet the contributors

Deborah Glover

Deborah Glover qualified in 1983 at University College Hospital, London. Clinical areas she has worked in include care of the elderly, oncology, ITU and HIV. Over the past few years she has been involved in practice and professional development roles and has brought her clinical and development experiences to her role as clinical editor for *Nursing Times*. Deborah's main passion is the development of practice that retains the values and principles of nursing.

Janet Hesketh

After spending several years trying to combine the roles of health visitor, Open University student, wife and mother, Janet moved into education full time to complete an MSc in Nursing. She joined the school of nursing, University of Wales, Bangor, in 1992 to teach behavioural science, nursing theory, social policy, and study skills to diploma and degree students and to develop further her own educational and research interests.

Phillip Hufton

Phillip is currently communications and development manager for the Thornbury Nursing Services Group. He has also been seconded as lead facilitator to the newly formed Federation of Independent Nursing Agencies. Prior to taking up that post, he worked in theatre recovery at the Countess of Chester NHS Trust, after successfully completing a Bachelor of Nursing Degree, at the University of Wales Bangor.

Whilst studying nursing, Phillip worked on the *Nursing Times* Student Steering Group, and wrote several pieces for *Nursing Times* and other publications. During his training he was an Active member of the RCN Association of Nursing Students, and Founding President of the Archimedes Society Students' Union.

Before his move into nursing, Phillip served as an army officer in various locations worldwide, and also worked for the government. During this time he successfully completed a degree in Management Science and Communication Studies and published a workbook on teambuilding and first level management. His hobbies include water-skiing, sailing, mountain sports, travel, popular cinema, music and cooking.

Student survival guide

Geoffrey Hunt

Geoffrey Hunt is senior lecturer in professional ethics at the University of Surrey and has edited four books in the field, including *Ethical Issues in Nursing* and *Whistleblowing in the Health Service*. He is assistant editor of the academic journal *Nursing Ethics*. Geoffrey is the founder of Freedom to Care, which supports whistleblowers and lobbies for greater corporate accountability. It may be contacted at PO Box 125, West Molesey, Surrey KT8 1YE.

Zosia Kmietowicz

Zosia Kmietowicz graduated from Liverpool University in 1986 with a BSc Hons in Pharmacology, and completed an MSc in Information Science at the City University in London two years later. She has been a freelance medical journalist for 10 years and contributes regularly to the medical and national consumer press.

Tony Makepeace

Tony Makepeace is currently a staff nurse on the Medical Directorate at Royal Preston Hospital. He qualified in April 1998 with a Diploma in Nursing from the University of Central Lancashire. Prior to that he obtained a BA (Hons) in history from the University of Manchester. While a student he was actively involved in student representation at the University, setting up a nationally distributed student magazine 'The Rubber Glove'. He has published articles in the past on student nursing and the period after qualifying. Interests include reading, swimming and Ipswich Town Football Club.

Jill Newman

Jill has been employed in the NHS since 1981 as a healthcare professional. Currently she manages two directorates within a combined acute and community trust, as well as having responsibility for risk management. Having completed professional qualifications in radiography, she proceeded to study health service management and obtained a first degree in economics and politics, followed by a Masters in Business Administration. In addition to her above role, Jill is heavily involved in the training of undergraduate students and lectures on organisational effectiveness. She also manages to find time to be a mother of two young children.

Mark Radcliffe

Mark Radcliffe MA, RMN, is mental health editor at Nursing Times. His hobbies include macrame, collecting spent matchsticks and practising a cool walk – but he does also want to save the planet and see world peace. His book, the *Seven Ages of Nursing*, gives the real lowdown on what it is like to be a student and post-registration nurse. It can be highly recommended because the acknowledgements include a thank you to the Banana Splits and Scooby Doo.

Martin Vousden

Martin Vousden, CDM and bar, is business manager of Nursing Times Projects, and now that he is an executive he has nothing to do with nursing or nurses. He tries to hide the fact that he trained as an RMN in Kent when Methuselah was a lad, and after 12 years in acute psychiatric nursing, in both hospitals and the community, he decided that journalism looked a much better option. Unfortunately this new career involved compiling a directory of healthcare information and resources, with over 2,300 entries, a small sample of which is represented in this book.

Eileen Walsh

Eileen joined the NHS in September 1994 as a graduate management trainee. She read chemistry at Queens University, Belfast, where she obtained a primary degree followed by an MSc in medical research. She is currently in the process of writing up her PhD thesis in medical research. As a graduate trainee with the NHS she studied for her postgraduate qualifications in health service management at the College of Medicine, University of Wales. Eileen is currently employed by the University Hospital, Birmingham, working directly for the Chief Executive in a corporate management role.

Introduction

Hello and welcome to the brave new world.

Over the next three or four years as you progress through your training, you will experience the ups and downs of all human (and some not so human) life. Mostly, it will not be easy, but mainly, whatever the situation, it will be rewarding. You will feel good about yourself, bad about yourself, and even indifferent at times. Be assured, however, that it is all worth it and there is light at the end of the tunnel!

If you have confidence in your ability (or can fool everyone into thinking you have), and give one hundred per cent to everything (apart from the end of a seven-night stretch), you will probably succeed. And when you succeed as a nurse, you will make a difference to people's lives.

Now, before you reach for the vomit bowl (usually cardboard or plastic, shaped like a kidney – a vomit bowl shaped organ, useful for filtering waste products or eating lightly fried on toast) just try telling people what you do as a career and watch their reaction. It won't be the same reaction that accountants get as they nibble vol-au-vents at a party.

Nursing has changed over the years, as have the people coming into nursing. It is no longer considered to be a vocation, it is now regarded as a profession. Nurses are no longer the doctors' handmaidens, although some of the more 'eminent' consultants haven't quite realised that and still persist in expecting us to know their glove size. However, nursing is still about comforting patients and their loved ones, although time constraints often push this particular nursing duty to the bottom of the list. We can offer serious clinical input, and assist in restoring a person's health, and/or well-being. We make a difference, not only in the physiological, but also in the psychological.

From our personal experience, it is nursing, and no other platform, that offers care, compassion, empathy and, above all, humanity, when it is needed the most, not only by those suffering directly, but also by those suffering as a result of those they love being sick and vulnerable, or dying.

Some say that nursing has lost its caring side. This, of course, is complete rubbish. We are well trained, well educated, autonomous practitioners at

Introduction

the 'sharp end' of patient care. You will encounter those who will view you as a threat. These people are just as likely to be of the Gary Glitter generation as of the Max Bygraves generation. The only ones who will accept you with equanimity are those who thought Duran Duran were a good idea. But don't worry, listen to your tutors, listen to your peers, and, above all, have faith in your own ability.

You will be put upon (and in some instances, put about), and you will be frustrated. But stick with it. Console yourself with a mantra such as 'the alternative is hairdressing, the alternative is hairdressing' and all will be well. Don't forget your humanity, and don't forget your caring. Many, many people really appreciate what you do rather than talking about how wonderful you are. These are the people who will offer what seem to be the smallest things, such as a kind word, a tender touch or a simple thank you. These make all the difference.

However, be assured nurse stereotyping still exists and you will experience it everywhere. If you are female, you will be a budding nymphomaniac; if you are male you will undoubtedly be a failed doctor or a sex maniac, probably both. Whether male or female people will say: 'Ah, a nurse. Isn't that nice... I don't know how you do it!' Just show them lots of gory pictures and say, 'Hurrah, works van' every time an ambulance goes past. They will soon realise that actually you have a sick mind and that suffering is ambrosia to you. And then will shut up.

So, welcome to your future. Welcome to one of the most rewarding, enduring, responsive and valuable, yet frustrating professions. Welcome to nursing.

Deborah Glover and Phillip Hufton
August 1999

1 The Getting of Wisdom
– a light-hearted introduction to student life

Mark Radcliffe

Hello, welcome, glad you could come. Now before you got here everyone spent about 20 years arguing about what kind of training we could offer you. We wanted something comprehensive, in keeping with the modern image of a modern profession. Something that included a sound clinical base, the personal development opportunities that would enable you to cope with the experiences and stresses that are so integral to the job. And the intellectual and academic skills to enable you to theorise effectively about nursing as a science while augmenting your critical skills, thus allowing you to make appropriate and informed clinical decisions. We also needed you to develop the human ability to comfort, reassure and inform your patients. To allow you to advocate on behalf of your patients, to communicate with them and with colleagues with equal ease and efficiency. We needed you to develop a vast range of technical skills and the wisdom to judge which of them is useful. Most importantly perhaps, we needed to offer you the emotional capacity to live in the stories of the people you work with. To hold hands with the dying, to listen, quietly, and know when or if or how to respond. We needed to offer you a training that would arm you, equip you to meet the avalanche of need you will face, and we want you to feel enabled, in 10 years' time to feel privileged, useful, wise and, most importantly, unbroken.

However we couldn't think of anything so you got Project 2000.

Student survival guide

Please don't be put off. Despite everything you may hear to the contrary, nurse training has always been more endurance test than well-planned educational opportunity. The fact that we all romanticise about our nurse training, despite how hellish it may have been, is because the experience was and always will be so powerful it's hard to let go of it. Sometimes maybe we feel threatened that that experience will be lost or undervalued and so we get protective. At other times we find ourselves believing in the way we practise and the foundations of that good practice, and imagine that is under threat. At yet other times we are afraid of what you might not know, forgetting all the things that we did not know. However, on other occasions, and let's be blunt about this, you are going to come across one or two bad apples that could spoil a good barrel. You should no more be put off by them than you should by the frailties of an education system that sometimes lets you down.

As a student you are going to have to endure many pointless things. There will be times on the wards when bored staff, anxious to prove to you that they have a sense of humour, will send you next door for 'a long stand' (geddit?). You will probably know that this is called a practical joke. However, you should know that you have three choices. You can go next door for a while, stand about a bit then come back and let them have their fun. Which is generous of you but means that a few days later they may send you off for a left handed syringe, the little pranksters. Or you can say cordially, 'I'm sorry but I do not believe in the long stand myth, please don't waste my time, I'm trying to nurse here,' which no matter how polite you are will gain you the reputation of being a smug know-it-all with no sense of humour. Or you could say, 'Sod off with the long stand gag you sad git,' which, while justified, may put a strain on your student-preceptor relationship.

While on the ward, if you are planning to be a general nurse there will be much talk about hats and stuff. This needn't be taken too seriously. It will essentially be just a precursor to the many conversations you will hear that will start with the words 'In my day…' as in, 'In my day we did proper nursing…', 'In my day we didn't have buses, we had to walk up to 20 miles a day just to do a shift and we wore our hats,' and 'In my day we didn't have fancy colleges, with your books and well-stocked fizzy drink dispensing machines, you lot don't know you're born.' Still, in fairness you will meet some people who nurse as well as Sinatra sang. For all the talk that surrounds your chosen profession, occasionally you see some work, or maybe do some work that makes you feel as though the planet you find yourself on finally fits. So don't worry about the long stand nonsense.

In the classrooms and lecture halls, of course, things can be different. The chances are some of the tutors are human, friendly, intelligent and supportive. But some of them are tossers. Imagine, if you are a woman, arriving at a party to find it filled with 15-year-old boys all desperate to impress you. They will not listen to anything you say, they will not ask you anything, and after drivelling on about nothing for about an hour they may try to persuade you to admire them by doing unsightly sit-ups on the carpet. If you don't clap or snog them they will call you names and maybe pull your hair. Well, some nurse tutors are a bit like that. They will often drivel on for hours but probably won't do the sit-ups. These are insecure people. Ignore them, they have no friends, they have come to education late and consider it something to be conquered rather then embraced. You can always tell a good teacher: s/he makes ideas understandable and accessible no matter how complex they are, because they want to share them in the hope that you will use them. No single idea in nursing is difficult to convey. If it sounds difficult it can only be because the teacher is a fool or he wants to impress you with his sit-ups. It is important that you do not take him seriously. Invent a stupid name for him; 'smudger' was popular in the 1950s, 'faceache' in the 1960s, but since then we have pretty much stuck with a 'dickhead' theme with a few variations according to any specific quality you may want to highlight.

One of the things you are likely to find as a student is that nursing is an activity steeped in a rich history of local and national myth. For example, my friend Victoria Blame tells of her first day on a medical ward, near the end of her training in a large London teaching hospital. She was shown round the fire exits, the intensive care beds, the kettle and finally – the sluice room. At this point her nurse guide began to look a little embarrassed and for the first time began to falter in instructions. Victoria, who is the Keeper of the Truth, quickly picked up on her new colleague's sudden discomfort and said:

'Shona, we have never met and to you I am a stranger but we are now colleagues and I hope one day friends. Now I sense that you are uncomfortable about something here but I know not what. Now Shona, I notice things and you may know that I am the Keeper of the Truth. I want you to tell me exactly what it is that is making you uncomfortable.'

'Why are you calling me Shona?'

Student survival guide

'Is that not your name, Shona?'

'No my name is Kevin.'

'I had no way of knowing.'

'Well, it's on my badge, and I am wearing trousers, and I introduced myself to you less than five minutes ago and I am married to your sister.'

'Oh yes it's coming back now,' said Victoria 'but I'm right in thinking there is something wrong am I not?'

'It's uncanny Victoria, you are right. I wish you'd noticed the whole boy-called-Kevin thing, but there you go. Your talents obviously lie elsewhere. Somewhere other than noticing the gender of the brother-in-law you work with…'

'Yes, yes get on with it,' said the Keeper of the Truth.

'Well it's about the sluice. It makes funny, sometimes embarrassing noises.'

'What sort of funny noises?'

'It's hard to describe…'

Victoria, having heard many a sluice, began to do impressions of sluices she has known, whirring and chugging away until she went quite pink. At this point the sister came in. Victoria was embarrassed, but needn't have been; the sister merely said:

'My, what an impressive array of sluice impressions. I can hardly wait for the Christmas party. What we would give for a sluice that made sounds like that. Can you do any other impressions? A horse maybe? Or Tommy Cooper?'

Victoria confirmed that she could indeed do a very fine impression of a horse and started cantering around the sluice room with Kevin on her back whinnying and clippety-clopping away like, well, a horse. Everyone was impressed but the sister quite rightly put a stop to the revelry and put the nurses back to work.

Later that evening Victoria, alone this time and a little tired, had to use the sluice for the first time. What was that sound? It was strange, eerie almost. And then she realised. The sluice whirred to the tune of 'Chattanooga Choo Choo' with barbershop quartet harmonies.

It appears that a member of a barbershop quartet had died on that ward almost 50 years ago and his colleagues, essentially a trio waiting to happen, had tried but failed to get to his bedside to pay their last respects. His dying wish was to hear, for one last time, 'Chattanooga Choo Choo' but he never did. And now every time the sluice is used that song reverberates around the ward.

This is just one example of nursing folklore. There are a million stories out there, some absurd, some spooky, most made up on tea breaks, but all an integral part of nursing. Take the story of Cathy Thyme.

A student nurse in the 1960s, Cathy was the sort of nurse who prompted the enviable comment, 'Oh she's got a lovely way with the patients, they all love her.' Some said Cathy was born to nurse. However she was dyslexic. In those days dyslexia attracted little sympathy or understanding and consequently many occasions arose that made her feel stupid. She was not stupid but she became insecure. The day before her finals an incident occurred on the drug round where Cathy was struggling with a long word and called for assistance. Under the circumstances this was a skilful and safe decision and because of it no drug error was made. However, a cruel junior doctor who looked a bit like Alec Baldwin and behaved like Terry-Thomas teased her mercilessly, calling her stupid and illiterate. She was neither but, in keeping with her background, her gender and the way of some nurses in those days, she felt stupid and illiterate.

The next day she attended her final exam. She was well equipped, she had pens and pencils, she even had a protractor. Of course nobody knows what a protractor is for but everyone takes one into exams in case they need it. More importantly she knew everything a student about to qualify needed to know and, with the words of the junior doctor ringing in her ears, she answered every question required, handed in her paper and tidied away her pencils and mathematical aids knowing that she had passed. Then she went back to her room in the nurses' home and hanged herself.

Legend has it, however, that this was not the end of Cathy's nursing career. A friend of mine who worked in the same hospital tells that on three separate occasions in the last 30 years when a young student nurse of much promise has struggled for reasons outside of her control, perhaps in the face of the stresses of the job or more commonly the thoughtless bullying of an arrogant medic, the ghost of Cathy Thyme appears. She rests a reassuring hand on the shoulder of the struggling nurse and, after waiting for an appropriate moment in the routine of the ward, she kicks seven bells out of the doctor.

Look out.

Student survival guide

In my day, training was based on the apprenticeship model. This essentially consisted of being thrown at wards and staff as early as possible and told to learn how to nurse by copying other nurses. It was a painful process. For apprenticeship models to work you pretty much need the Yoda method, I think. That is, you the student nurse need to be paired with some green eared muppet with all the answers, who will teach you to nurse like a space warrior. However, in reality you tended to get given whoever was not on duty when the charge nurse asked the question, 'So who wants the next student then?' As you changed wards every three months your learning experience was down to chance. In practice it was a bit of a disaster.

However, in principle at least, and if you were lucky and quite determined, there was a bit of an education in there that could be squeezed out. The simple priority of being with patients and learning from them was clear. However, we were forced to confront our own ignorance a dozen times a day in what was often a hostile environment. One of the big pluses was the fact that we trained in small, easy to store groups of about 15. Usually at least three people dropped out so about a dozen of us spent three years together and we got to know each other quite well. I trained in one of the old, now long defunct 'bins'. We started with six weeks in what was then called 'school' and then we were thrown at the elderly mentally ill back-wards and left there for three months. Apparently this was done because the powers that be felt that if you were going to be driven out by the hopelessness in the walls of those old spiteful asylums it would save money and time to get you out early.

We were encouraged to use our group as a major form of support, which we did. We learnt to nurse in much the same way as you I suspect, by sitting around getting drunk, howling at the moon and comparing horror stories. We swore we would be better than what we saw, and never indulge ourselves with pointless confrontation. Our training in that environment was an exercise in developing strategies for change. We took comfort from each other's outrage and anger, and plotted ways of making tiny alterations. My first was to try to make sure that demented old ladies were never fed while they were defecating. A small thing perhaps but it seemed a good place to make a stand. Our stands were like signatures, proving to ourselves we had been in this timeless place and had left a mark of sorts. Such was our romance.

Frankly it was all terribly emotional, a bit like a Bette Davis film. Perhaps we were pathetic. All clean and righteous. Surrounded by staff who had been there longer than the patients. But it is, I suspect, a history shared by some of the staff who irritate you now. I think the reality is that the problem you are forced to endure is a clash of cultures. Yours is different to ours.

And let's not imagine that in the world of general nursing things were wonderful either. Victoria Blame trained in the olden days when dance music was called 'disco' and Spandau Ballet happened.

She reports that on her first ward, after a mere six weeks, she was repeatedly sent by the senior staff nurse to whom she was assigned to 'prepare the trolley for a chest drip' or to 'resite and set the saline'. Thus Victoria was forced to spend all day saying she did not know how to do that and be treated as a fool. She tells how the wards then were not really focused on patients but instead on routines. She herself was once strongly reprimanded by a sister for wheeling a trolley to a bedside, in preparation for doing a dressing, but committing the heinous crime of taping the disposal bag to the trolley in such a way as to appear unsymmetrical. Her punishment? She had to do 50 press-ups and swear never to tape anything to a trolley without using a protractor again. It was important that the students learnt in those days that the wheels of a trolley when stationary had to all face the same direction.

She tells also of one of her first ward rounds when the God known as consultant arrived on the ward and began to pronounce on the sick. Irritatingly one of the patients was having a shave at the time of the great man's arrival, so the consultant marched to the semi-bearded patient and, without saying a word, unplugged the electric razor before returning to take centre stage. No nurse did a thing, although later another student, to his eternal credit, complained at the handover that this was no way to treat the patients and that surely we, the nurses, should be stopping this sort of pomposity. He was threatened with dismissal. This was in 1987. Not 1895.

It's worth remembering that the same nurses who tell you that everything used to be better, and that patient care always came first, often trained under these circumstances. In a climate of fear, the activity of nursing was a series of tasks; patients were occasionally irritating distractions from the routine of the ward. In the same way perhaps that human beings are the bane of an architect's life, patients were sometimes the fly in the otherwise aseptic ointment of ward life. My friend Rita Blood cried every night for a month when she started nursing. Not because of the suffering she saw but

Student survival guide

because of the nonsense she had to endure to become a nurse. I don't imagine that for one second, when you as a student are taking nonsense in whatever form you may find it, you can take comfort from the fact that nonsense is some kind of hereditary arrangement in nursing. But it may do no harm to de-romanticise the whole 'in my day we did proper nursing' rubbish. A lot of people did, but a lot more polished stuff, deferred to unthinking medics and made the students' lives a misery.

I asked Rita how she coped and she says, as many people do, that she came across one or two people who inspired her. Romance again? Probably not. Rita tells of working on an elderly unit with terribly institutionalised, unthinking staff with long and poorly formed habits. Apparently a newly arrived sister, who came to nursing late but with an energy and enthusiasm that put her younger colleagues to shame, set out to challenge some of the less savoury elements of care. For example, was it really necessary to prepare the patients for bed at four o'clock in the afternoon and make sure they had all retired, after toileting, by five? One suspects not unless they all had a paper round to get up for. And why was it that none of the patients ever left the ward? This woman started arranging trips to the shops, to the seaside; she changed the ward routine as best she could.

A few years later Rita met the nice lady again doing agency work with the district nurses. She was planning to take early retirement; she had lost weight and faith. Her staff had stopped talking to her and she had found a dead mouse in her desk drawer three days in a row. Mouse flu suggested her staff? She left. Things went back to normal.

Things weren't better in those days. In fact things were crap. What was better perhaps was that the lines between doing your job well and doing it badly were clearer. The possibility of doing a good thing in the face of the bad was greater. The struggle was simple if sometimes seemingly impossible. And like people remember the ugliness of wars with a sense of misplaced glee then some nurses recall their struggles because they were life affirming.

Part of the rationale for Project 2000 was to protect students from that rubbish and to sterilise and perhaps dignify the process of learning to nurse. I would applaud that but, and I realise I should apologise for this, I hope you have your battles too. I hope you see things that make the blood course through your veins and you change them, slightly, fret about them healthily, because that is the role of a student nurse whether it's written into the curriculum or not.

Nursing now exists in a post-modern age and is not afraid to prove it. A lot of nonsense is imagined about what post-modernism means. Which is of course a trick; it doesn't actually mean anything. It is loosely just a label to mark the end of thinking about things in the way that we have always tended to think about things. Primarily it imagines that absolute philosophical truths no longer exist. It presupposes that history has finished and that God is dead and most importantly – and this is the bit I like best – all cultural activity must be equal. Primarily, perhaps, because the systems of value and meaning that are attached by habit or prejudice or taste are rendered empty. So Mozart is no more significant or worthy than that 'Shake and Vac' advert. So why am I boring you with a crass bastardisation of modern thought? (Like I can remember any of this stuff.) Well obviously it's an overlong build up to a stupid story.

As a student nurse you are entering a confusing world. Because as I said earlier you are going to be gently teased and have crass practical jokes done near and to you, you may come to doubt many things you hear regardless of how intelligent you are. My friend Rita has been nursing for 13 years. She has run units, worked independently in the voluntary sector and in primary care. She has a degree in law, which she took part time because she wanted to be stimulated by something other than nursing. She has a Master's degree in organisation psychology. I don't know why she did that; I think she wanted to organise stuff. She currently works as a health visitor. However, on her first ward while training she received a seemingly ridiculous circular sent to all the new nurses and to this day, and despite herself, she cannot quite decide if it was somebody's idea of a joke or if it was serious. Such is the strange world of nursing.

The circular said: 'All female nurses are instructed to wear tights. Stockings are not permitted in this hospital. This is because of the infection control implications of pubic fallout.'

It is quite probable that they were serious. Indeed most general nurses of around my age say they experienced the same thing. But how was it to be checked? And by whom?

I imagine that a large part of your experience, which separates you from all the nurses who trained before you, is the relationship you have with the new universities. I don't envy you this. Quite simply in the past, pre-Thatcher certainly, when people went to university (or polytechnic as they were often called in the olden days) it was to read interesting books and have sex with unlikely people. Of course you picked up a degree but the process became more important than the goal and the goal tended to be,

Student survival guide

for a lot of people at least, vague and unfocused. Real world things like nursing were too important for the universities and the universities were too self-absorbed and sober and formal to concern themselves with such realities. Obviously there were 'vocational' courses available but they were in things like engineering and business studies and nobody spoke to the people who did things like that.

Now of course you are between a rock and a hard place. The credibility gap punishes you and there is little you can do about it except find a way to spit in the eye of the snobs and curse the insecure fools who play into the hands of tradition by trying to constantly 'prove' that they and nursing are academically worthy. You are in a poverty trap and may find it hard to enjoy the social setting of university because often nursing is stuck in a small off-campus college away from other students. You may find you share bits of courses with social scientists, which must be vile, and biological scientists, which must be dull. And when they get long school-like holidays and take their washing home to parents you get sent to do something like work in some sort of hospital or health care setting where you may find you are not always greeted with open arms.

Perhaps one of the most disgusting and frustrating limits that comes with the 'special status' that accompanies nurse education in the universities is the strange thing known as a bursary.

Yes, it's a little more than a grant but God help you if you get ill or break a limb or some other misfortune. You will have your bursary stopped. You will not get any sick pay, you cannot sign on because you will have to leave your course and you cannot go to the hardship fund because it won't cover illness. You are, and I choose my words carefully here, buggered.

It's all well and good trying to attract people into nursing but as soon as you get here you realise the welfare rights they are afforded are apparently modelled on the system designed by the same bloke who designed the woollen swimsuit. And I don't mean that in a good way. In fact the administration of your student experience does, from the outside, look remarkably similar to a woollen swimsuit – full of holes and difficult to iron. Here we are crying out for new nurses, mourning the lack of new recruits, anxiously trying to attract people in spite of the crises of morale and terrible wages, and it would appear that all the training places are full with a massive overflow of applicants and nowhere for them to go. Still, no doubt our greatest nursing minds are on the case and we can expect somebody to round up the usual suspects, form a sub-committee, give them a grant, a nice room with biscuits and ask them to urgently come up with a solution (more training opportunities perhaps? Sorry I'm guessing) and to have it written up in draft form for the civil service by 2023 at the latest.

Sorry about the state of things, it's one of the problems with social experimentation, because for all the planning and good intentions it's down to you to make it work.

Another significant problem is the fact that you may feel baseless. The university is not quite home, particularly if you are in an isolated college and they may have contracts with about 154 different clinical environments. You are always a visitor, always passing through. Wherever you lay your hat, that's your head; another town another hotel room. You are like Clint Eastwood was in those spaghetti westerns, always moving from town to town, doing good, maybe shooting Eli Wallach. You are the stranger in town. And while we are swimming around in cultural references do you remember that song called 'I've been to Paradise but I've never been to me'? No reason, just wondered.

The universities get more money per head for you than for any other student. So it's reasonable to expect little presents from the tutors and the administrators, just as a way of them thanking you for your efforts and for your choosing to be a nurse. Everyone benefits from you making the choice you have made: the profession, the universities, the patients, the state, the companies that make nursing accessories. No doubt someone will give you a list at some point, outlining all the accessories that you or your parents must buy for you. Whoever gives you the list probably has shares in the company. You will think it odd that you don't get all this stuff for free so think carefully when you look at the list. Do you really need all this stuff?

Uniforms, fob watch, books, belt, several pairs of practical pants, tights, sensible shoes, maybe so. But do you need the special nurse whistle? Or the special nurse moped with 'I'm a nurse' painted on the side? Do you need your own thermometer or stethoscope? I don't think you do. Mental health nurses, do you need even one sociology book? Of course not. And put back that special nurse chocolate cake, it's not an essential tool of your trade. And don't pay for those handouts in lectures or from the library either; how many times are you supposed to have to pay for your education?

Nursing often attracts a more mature student. Some of them can be really, really old, like 22. Often even older. This is a good thing but for the mature student it can be an added responsibility. Apart from the fact that you older ones will feel obliged to listen to a whole range of personal issues from fellow students from all kinds of courses, including homesickness, sexual identity, sexual inadequacy, never having had sex, having just had sex and not knowing who is supposed to apologise first, having figured out, post-sex, who has to apologise but not knowing who should pick the pizza. Then there's unrequited love, getting first-time drunks home without them throwing up on you and existential angst. (This last is compulsory by the way. It is the law that during your university days you have to ask yourself what the point of everything is loads of times and sigh hopelessly because nobody understands what a sensitive soul you are.) You will play parent and consequently you may not be given permission to play at the student parties. Well I suggest you play and be damned. If you want to drink crème de menthe from the trouser pocket of the senior lecturer go right ahead. The good thing about being mature is that most things you do that are in fact ridiculous look quite cool to the young. Take the crème de menthe thing for example. Go ahead, sip away, unless said educator is wearing cords obviously because they can feel a bit coarse round the lip I gather, but otherwise sip away, the kids will think it's some kind of rock and roll thing.

It is more than possible of course that you may have grown-up commitments like family and thus any hope of 'living the student experience' is perhaps limited. It is said that being a mature entrant in nursing is something of a two-edged sword. However I can't comment on that because I have no idea what it means. Can you have a one-edged sword? Or a four-edged sword, which one imagines is basically a long square lump of metal with a handle... anyway. On the one hand if you are a mature entrant you are likely to have many life skills that you bring to the training. You may have actually had other jobs, you may have been a health care assistant or a civil servant or a swimming instructor or a paperboy. All of these things will equip you for your future in nursing with the possible exception of swimming instructor, although having said that if there's a flood you will be the one your colleagues rely on. Have you ever seen the Poseidon Adventure? That bit where a plump Shelley Winters does the underwater swimming? If you are nursing on an overturned cruise ship in the middle of the ocean your pre-nursing life could come into its own.

The down side is you may not be used to the language and convention of modern study. You will of course get used to it, but in the meantime enjoy not knowing. In the research methods class talk of your commitment to 'evidence-based rashes' and 'random patrol trials'. When they tell you that you are expected to write a long essay before qualifying ask them 'how long does the end of course vivisection have to be?'. When they shout 'dissertation', say 'bless you'.

In the main you may find yourself feeling the strangest things during your training, from rage and despair to compulsion and profound if sometimes unfocused satisfaction. For all the supposed reductionism of nursing and the twee professionalisation, what you are going to be doing for as long as you do it will bring you as close or closer to the nature of things than any other activity. Enjoy, and if all that silly unnecessary essay writing bugs you, don't worry, it has sod all to do with nursing. In the words of the once lovely David Bowie, obviously before his Tin Machine days: 'If the homework gets you down throw the books on the fire and we'll take the car down town.' Give us a call; I have a car.

2 The Way We Were
– the history of nursing

Marsh Gelbart

Too often the history of nursing is distilled down to a tale of great innovators, leaders and reformers with Florence Nightingale to the fore. The story of nursing is presented as a seamless progression. Yet the narrative is more complex and messy than this. An alternative perspective of nursing history reveals certain trends: poor pay and conditions, second rate training and an obsession with uniforms and hierarchy. Status has been mistaken for professionalism and having a vocation has been substituted for adequate financial remuneration.

The evolution of nursing has been influenced by class and gender. The position of women in society and the history of nursing are interrelated. The nursing profession in Victorian Britain grew up in a deeply paternalistic era, against a background of a society stratified and segmented by class and gender. Anxieties around female sexuality also had an influence. Given these factors, it is no wonder that female subordination in society as a whole was mirrored in the caring professions (Macfarlane, 1990).

CHAOS, CLASS AND CONTRADICTIONS

Nursing the sick is a function that has occurred since humans formed communities. More often than not, care of the sick was undertaken by women. The first organised nursing was associated with the religious orders. However, what we recognise as nursing in the modern sense evolved in the 19th century.

During this time, industrialisation saw the growth of great urban conurbations. The population increase overwhelmed the existing hospital system. Voluntary hospitals were set up to meet the demands of a burgeoning population, supplementing hospitals that had existed since medieval times. An under-funded system, based within the workhouses, came into existence alongside the voluntary hospitals. The workhouses not only housed the desperate poor, they also provided basic care for sick inmates. Poor-law nursing was a form of domestic service carried out by able-bodied females interned within the grim confines of the workhouse. To the Victorians, poverty was almost considered a form of disease.

Nurses who worked prior to the reforms of the mid-19th century, not just those who plied their trade in the workhouses, had negligible training. Conditions of service were poor. So much so that nursing staff supplemented their miserable wages by stealing from the patients and were over fond of alcohol (Clark-Kennedy, 1962).

Scientific advances in the latter part of the 19th century revolutionised medicine's understanding of disease and allowed advances in treatment. In order to cope with the increasingly technical demands of patient care, there grew a need for more and better nurses who had undergone formal, secular training.

There had been isolated initiatives abroad. In 1798 at New York Hospital, Dr Valentine Seaman had introduced a series of medical lectures tailored for the needs of nursing staff. And in 1859 a training school for nurses was established at Lausanne, Switzerland (Deloughery, 1977).

In Britain there had been some reforms, but they lacked a clear secular orientation. In 1848 a school that combined nurse training with religious and moral discipline was set up at St John's House, London. St John's House took over nurse training at King's College Hospital. These measures lacked the impact of the reform process introduced by Florence Nightingale in the wake of the Crimean war of 1854–56.

Nightingale's reforms were instigated after her experiences in the Crimea. She made her reputation fighting the administrative chaos that hindered the care of the wounded. At the barrack hospital at Scutari, Nightingale and a band of nursing sisters laid down the foundations of modern nursing – for good and for ill.

Mary Seacole, a contemporary of Nightingale, also worked in the Crimea. Born in Jamaica in 1805, Seacole had experience of tending patients with yellow fever and other diseases. Her offer of help at Scutari was rejected. Unlike Nightingale, Seacole worked under the burden of having the wrong class background and skin colour. Nonetheless, she earned an enviable reputation for providing nursing and medical care for soldiers at the front. Her interventions complimented Nightingale's organisational skills (Kelsey, 1998).

In the aftermath of the Crimea, in 1860, Nightingale founded the school of nursing at St Thomas' Hospital. Here probationer nurses undertook a one-year training regime, which borrowed some aspects of its behaviour from religious orders. The school opened its doors to respectable, motivated women of all social backgrounds. While previously the majority of nursing staff had been made up working class women, now entrants from privileged backgrounds enlisted into training. Nightingale wished to synthesise the hardiness of working class probationers with the education and 'breeding' of the lady entrants. All were expected to be of a high moral standing.

Nightingale's system saw the development of a coherent body of nursing behaviour. The nurse probationers worked in a tightly disciplined structure, subordinate to the wishes of the matron. They carried out duties requested by the medical staff, but translated through matron's understanding of those wishes. In turn the matron, and Nightingale herself, had to fight against the obstructive attitudes of many doctors, who felt that the new nurses were impinging on their profession.

The new model of nursing involved a number of contradictory aspects. Nurses were responsible for the cleanliness of the wards and patients, but were regarded as more than mere domestics. Nurses carried out aspects of care, such as dressing wounds, which had once been the domain of the medical students. Yet they were considered less than a doctor. Nursing had established its existence as a separate body. It had status, but had yet to develop any real autonomy.

By 1900 only 982 nurses had been trained at the original Nightingale school (Baly, 1983). Of 25,000 trained nurses at the turn of the century, only 10,000 had been through Nightingale-style training (Hart, 1994). However, their ideas and aspirations dominated, particularly among those nurses who worked in the voluntary hospitals. They saw themselves as an elite.

Some nurses saw registration as a guarantor of autonomy and consolidator of status. Ethel Bedford Fenwick, an ex-matron of St. Bartholomew's Hospital, London, led the drive for nurse registration. This would prevent anyone who had not been formally trained as a nurse from acting as one. However, she also believed that nurse probationers should receive no payment, and should pay for the privilege of training in order to reserve nursing as exclusively a profession of 'women of breeding'. Bedford Fenwick partially succeeded – in 1919 nursing became registered. However, entry to nurse training remained free. This established a form of elitism which relied on training rather than breeding (Hart, 1994).

In the 1930s, nursing suffered a recruitment crisis. Consequently a second, less academic, route into nursing, State Enrolment, became available. Similarly in the 1950s, a chronic shortage of nurses allowed males into general nursing.

Until the second decade of the 20th century male nurses were largely consigned to asylum work. Treatment and care followed a pattern of containment rather than cure. The predominantly male nursing staff, often working in grimmer environments than general nurses, worked as poorly trained attendants. What reform there was came about through rank and file trade union activity, rather than pressure from the Nightingale trained nursing elite (Carpenter, 1980).

FROM RITUAL TO RESEARCH

If nursing was dependent on training to accentuate its status, how good was the instruction provided?

As medicine became able to treat a wide spectrum of illnesses, so nurses required ever more complex technical skills. As nurses became responsible for the monitoring of a patient's condition, they had less time to carry out some of the aspects of nursing connected to Nightingale's reforms. Domestic functions, such as ensuring ward hygiene, were transferred from the nurses to hospital cleaners.

Yet the quality of the training required for the more demanding role failed to keep pace. 'The greatest obstacle to change was the apprenticeship system of training, which in nursing persisted long after other skilled and semi-skilled occupations transferred the burden of training to the formal education institutions of the state.' (Castle, 1983) Nursing was failing to keep up with the educational standards of other professions, while the technical skills demanded of the nurse were expanding.

In essence, nurses were being trained rather than educated. Training was too often done by rote, was inflexible and led to the retention of ritualistic procedures for patient care (Ford and Walsh, 1994). Training had the 'advantage' of providing a regular supply of student and pupil nurses on a ward, where they constituted a pool of 'cheap labour'. However, the rapid turnover of trainees on the ward was not conducive to patient care or quality of nurse education. Procedures, patriarchy, duty, discipline, ritual and routine were the warp and weft of nurse training until recent years.

Today, nurse education based on theory, research and questioning is the norm. Degree-based courses have supplanted the old ward-based apprenticeships. Patient-centred, flexible, knowledge-based nursing methodologies are now, at least on paper, prevalent. However, restricted resources, low staffing levels on the wards and increased workloads have taken away the gloss from the new system. In some ways, the supplementing of a restricted number of qualified nurses by a larger number of dedicated but untrained and underpaid ward assistants is a retrograde step.

POVERTY PAY

Nursing has traditionally been an undervalued and underpaid occupation. In part this has been as a consequence of it being a predominantly female calling, portrayed as a vocation, with nurses reluctant to take industrial action. A brief overview of the wages of nurses over the years and the comparative pay of other workers makes for interesting reading.

In the 1820s the head nurse of the London Hospital earned five guineas a year. Ward nurses earned from four guineas down to one guinea. The hospital carpenter earned a princely £7 17s 6d (Clark-Kennedy, 1962). At St Thomas' Hospital in the 1880s, a clear distinction was drawn between women of working class backgrounds and ladies of breeding. All underwent identical nursing training. Yet working class women would rarely be expected – or allowed – to progress beyond the grade of staff nurse earning between £18 and £30 a year. The ladies on the other hand, would expect to earn £35 to £60 a year as sisters. By 1890 an ordinary cook earned £35 a year, but a trained nurse could expect £25 (Helmstadter, 1997).

In 1897 the records of the Wages Board at Lancaster County Asylum showed that the highest paid attendant received £40 a year. Most asylum day nurses, who were male, earned between £16 and £22 a year. A contemporary police constable after eight years service earned £75 a year, a female weaver £37, and a male engineering fitter £83 (Carpenter, 1980).

Low pay has not been limited to the 19th century. In 1937 British nurses took part in an unprecedented march. Masked to prevent identification and resultant disciplinary action, several hundred nurses demonstrated against long hours, low wages and staffing shortages. In 1937, a staff nurse took home £60 to £80 a year – well below the level of female workers in less demanding jobs.

In 1970 a student nurse took home between £6 and £7 a week. A staff nurse earned £18 a week; considerably lower than the national average. Work patterns often involved split shifts and there was no automatic additional payment for night shifts or weekend work (Widgery, 1979). Nationwide unrest in 1971 helped nurses to obtain reasonable pay increases. Nevertheless, poor pay continued. In 1987 a nurse's average wage was £7,800. That of a policeman was £13,500. A student nurse earned some £5000 less than a probationary policeman (Hart, 1994).

In the early 1990s, a newly qualified staff nurse earned 16% less than a newly qualified policewoman. To rub salt in the wound, a newly qualified staff nurse earned some 30% less than a person starting work behind a bank counter (Hart, 1994).

APPALLING ACCOMMODATION

Accommodation provided for nurses has always been a topic for heated discussion. 'The first nurses often lived out, probably in the adjacent slums. Towards the end of the 18th century, they tended to live in. No doubt the governors felt they could control them better that way.' (Baly, 1977). At St John's House the nurses of 'high breeding' slept in separate bedrooms. Meanwhile working class nurses slept in cubicles crowded in dormitories (Helmstadter, 1997).

In 1869 the Times correspondent described the living quarters at Bart's Hospital, where the probationary nurses were obliged to live, as 'a disgrace to humanity'. At Bart's (and other hospitals), strict control was kept over the social life and sexual behaviour of nurses in residence. Well into the 1930s, nurses not on duty had to be in their rooms by 10 in the evening, with lights out half an hour later (Yeo, 1995). Of course, male visitors were not allowed in the residences. Until recent years many nurses continued to live in sub-standard hospital accommodation. This is no longer the case. As trusts have sold off property including residences, low paid nurses have moved back to the adjacent slums. Progress at last!

STATUS AND SCIATICA

Nurses' lives remained, until recent years, circumscribed by petty rules (and some would argue they still are). Many of these regulations, which were of a hideous complexity, pertained to uniform codes (Yeo, 1995). The reasons why are instructive. Discipline was seen as necessary, to bring order from the chaos that pre-dated Nightingale's reforms. Consequently, nursing adopted some of the mindset of the military that helped to create a very hierarchical structure. This was reflected in nuances of nursing dress and symbols of rank and seniority.

At first glance nurses' uniforms merely fulfil a number of pragmatic functions. These include the ready identification of role and rank, while allowing the nurse to perform a number of demanding physical tasks. However, nursing outfits also carry a psychological meaning: they demonstrate commitment and dedication. For many nurses, uniforms impart a sense of professionalism and status. Unfortunately psychology, aesthetics and status have too often outweighed ergonomics and practicality.

In 1996 an Institute of Employment Studies report identified nursing as the second highest risk occupation for musculo-skeletal conditions. Over half of all work-related illnesses among nurses are back-related (Gates, 1997).

CONCLUSION

The history of British nursing is complex. Although there have been singular reformers and innovators who have shaped the pattern of nursing, their contribution cannot be taken in isolation. Social factors, such as the position of women in society, class structure and the struggle of rank and file nurses to better their conditions, have also moulded modern nursing. Repeated patterns of poor pay and conditions of service will continue to exist until nurses learn from their past.

References

Baly, M. (1977) *Nursing*. London: Batsford Ltd.

Baly, M. (1983) The Nightingale Nurses: The myth and the reality. In: Maggs, C. (ed.) *Nursing History: The State of the Art*. Wolfeboro, New Hampshire: Croom Helm.

Carpenter, M. (1980) Asylum nursing before 1914: A chapter in the history of labour. In: Davies, C. (ed.). *Rewriting Nursing History*. London: Croom Helm.

Castle, J. (1983) The development of professional nursing in New South Wales, Australia. In: Maggs, C. (ed.). *Nursing History: The State of the Art*. Wolfeboro, New Hampshire: Croom Helm.

Clark-Kennedy, A.E. (1962) *The London: A Study in the Voluntary Hospital System*. London: Pitman Medical Publishing Company.

Deloughery, G. (1977) *History and Trends in Professional Nursing*. St Louis, Missouri: The C.V. Mosby Company.

Ford, P., Walsh, M. (1994) *New Rituals for Old*. London: Butterworth Heinemann.

Gates, E. (1997) Handling problems. *Health and Safety*; 19: 6, 9–12.

Hart, C. (1994) *Behind the Mask: Nurses, their Unions and Nursing Policy*. London: Bailière Tindall.

Helmstadter, C. (1997) Doctors and nurses in the London teaching hospitals: class, gender, religion and professional expertise, 1850–1890. *Nursing History Review*; 5, 161–197.

Kelsey, J. (1998) The Black Nightingale. *Meditheme*; 17: 4, 101–102.

Macfarlane, M.E. (1990) The professional nurse: with or without a uniform. *Canadian Journal of Nursing Administration*; 3: 3, 14–17.

Widgery, D. (1979) *Health in Danger: The Crisis in the National Health Service*. London: Macmillan Press Ltd.

Yeo, G. (1995) *Nursing at Bart's*. Stroud, Glos.: Alan Sutton Publishing Limited.

3 Being There – preparation for theory and practice

Erica Forth

It is probably safe to assume that if you are reading this you are about to start, or are contemplating undertaking, some form of nurse education, be it a diploma or degree, and are wondering what to expect and how you should be feeling about it.

BE AFRAID, VERY AFRAID!

It is very difficult to generalise about what to expect from nurse education. That sounds like a cop out but unfortunately it's true. Everyone's experience is individual; everyone gets something different out of it. There is one absolute 'dead cert' – whatever sort of person you are now, you will be a different one by the end.

Of course, what you are about to embark on is no journey paved with gold, or silver, and for that matter coppers will be few and far between. However, if you are looking for a job that can be indescribably satisfying, thrilling and meaningful; if you want a job that will provide you with endless entertaining anecdotes to repulse the population of your local pub; and if you want the right to enter 'smug mode' at many a social gathering, as people gaze upon you in awe muttering phrases like, 'Oh, I could never do it', then you might just have picked the right job.

GREAT EXPECTATIONS (NOT)

On the first day of your first placement, you don't need to know it all – nobody will expect you to. And although you shouldn't be out of your depth and you are unlikely to cause much damage, you should be prepared to face the old chestnut of 'don't they teach you anything in school anymore' and a small fountain of equally derogatory remarks about today's nurse education.

Thankfully, you are unlikely to find yourself spending hours in classes learning how to do 'hospital corners' and theatre beds. Gone are the days of sitting in groups, learning how to take each other's blood pressure. There will, however, be lectures on why a bed should be made properly and what crumpled up sheets can do to a delicate derrière, with the research to prove what you are being taught. Expect to collect huge amounts of research papers on everything you can possibly think of; expect to be taught to question and think, not be told and just do.

You should not expect to:

- take charge of the ward;
- cover for staff shortages or sickness;
- work unsupervised;
- do things you are not happy to do;
- work ten weekends in a row;
- be used as a general dogsbody while on placement.

I list these examples in the strong hope that there are no longer any places that treat nursing students in this way, but I am realistic enough to know that at least some of these practices still occur.

As far as teaching goes, you can expect to be a part of a large university, and yes, you can even wear your own clothes to lectures. There are very few tutors now who are not well qualified and highly experienced.

Don't expect worksheets, homework and tutors breathing down your neck if you start to fall behind. Do expect to get used to the phrases 'self directed learning' and 'you are all adult learners now'. Don't expect right and wrong answers to every question. There are no set texts any more; answers are only as right as the research that backs them up suggests. If you can prove with research that black could be suggested to be white, then a good nurse you will make.

There are, one has to say, very few things in the social arena of nurse education that we are not thankful have gone. There is no longer a curfew at the nurses' home. Don't expect some scary matron to hijack you in the corridors for being late/drunk/with company, but on the other hand she won't be there to wake you up when you sleep in either.

As far as clinical issues are concerned, as long as you go in with a reasonably realistic point of view, you shouldn't get too many nasty shocks. Although you can expect to be assessed by highly competent, knowledgeable people, sadly you can't always expect to find that they are motivated, enthusiastic or even happy in their work. You are entering a profession that is in the midst of a whirlwind of change, and nobody is entirely comfortable with change. You are entering a profession that in many cases feels undervalued, underpaid and downtrodden.

You can expect at some point in your training to come across professionals who feel threatened by your generation, whether it is because you come out with a higher qualification than them, or simply because you are younger and fresher than they are.

You can expect to be told that you are wasting your time, that nursing isn't a profession worth working for. All I can say is that only those who are in it can change it, and only those who truly care will make any difference. Nobody said it was going to be easy, but nobody said it wasn't worth it either.

In terms of your education don't expect:

- to be treated like any other student in the university. Universities have only recently taken over nurse education and they haven't quite got their heads round it yet. Most degree students go home for the holidays. The universities cater for this timetable by closing down services during summer, Easter and Christmas;
- permanent residences (universities fundraise by emptying halls of residence of students to hire them out to tourists and conferences).

Prepare to become a minority during the holidays. Some universities are beginning to provide basic facilities for nursing students: essentials such as occupational health, library facilities, even a certain amount of catering and social input is available to the chosen few. But if you are in need of a student union officer, you may find that s/he'll be away on training/on holiday/back at the start of term.

Don't expect lots of MONEY. If you decide on the degree route, then prepare for student loans, overdrafts and, when you qualify, graduate loans to pay off overdrafts. If you choose to take the diploma programme to reach your goal then you will be paid... a pittance. You will be lucky if you manage to find a bank that will give you student terms. You are not entitled to student loans, you are unlikely to be entitled to hardship funds and you can't get a regular part time job because you work shifts. You will be lucky if you manage to get a graduate loan at the end and, on top of this, all the other students in the university will think you're rolling in it!

REALISTIC EXPECTATIONS

As far as clinical experience is concerned, I can almost guarantee that provided you go in with a positive and keen attitude, you will have some great experiences and learn almost more than the average brain can take in. Be prepared first of all to learn a whole new language – the language of medical terminology. This will include the most bizarre abbreviations and words that would tickle even the dullest of imaginations.

Chances are you will spend the first few months making a proverbial prat of yourself until you get the hang of it, but this comes with the territory, and every nurse around you will take pleasure in telling you about the time when it happened to them. It's like being initiated into a club. When you get in – which will happen quicker than you think – you will do exactly the same thing to the next student behind you. It's the first thing that you get to pass on, and it will feel good.

You can definitely expect to come across some amazing nurses, some that would have put Florence Nightingale herself to shame. You will have the honour of watching nurses with unending patience and compassion, no matter what circumstances they are working under. You will see acts of kindness and thoughtfulness that stun you. You can expect to find nurses whose time is under pressure, but who always find time for you. There are still many nurses who understand the importance of good student experiences and will bend over backwards to help and support you. This could be explaining a simple procedure to you for the hundredth time that day without a hint of displeasure, or taking you out for a pint on your last shift with them.

Student survival guide

Nurses are genuinely good people, and most take great pleasure in teaching and sharing knowledge. We can all remember what it was like to be a student. Overall, nurses recognise that you are the future of their profession and so want to nurture and support you as much as possible. There may be different reasons for it: some will feel they want to give you the skills you need, some think that it is simply part of their role as a nurse and some really enjoy teaching. As long as they teach you well, what does it matter what the motive is.

On the wards you can expect to face a thousand emotions as you witness a whole spectrum of events, from birth to death, from the trauma of an accident to the joys of a cure, from successful treatment to a peaceful end from suffering. You can expect to be overjoyed one shift and devastated the next. You can expect to be allowed access to the most private aspects of people's lives. You will be trusted, for no other reason than the fact that you wear a uniform. You will be expected to become immune to what you see; you may feel that you have to become hard and tough. If you manage to do that, then tell us your secret, because if you care enough to be a nurse, then the events that you see will always affect you, and one patient now and then will always get to you.

Not all you are taught will make sense, but surprisingly most of it finds some relevance eventually. You can expect to be taught by some very good tutors and you will probably find one in particular whose style suits you and who you can relate to. You can expect that the best support often comes from your peers. I can remember many theories becoming as clear as day once discussed in the pub after class.

Social life as a nursing student may be difficult, but never impossible! Money will be a problem, but agency work and cheap nights out are the key. The bonus side of the higher education setting is, of course, the student bar. Here's an insider tip: become a student rep for your student union – you will get bought pints for it.

If you want to be a nurse, be prepared to put up with the bad bits. Tears, tantrums, traumas and triumphs will be a part of your everyday life, so if you can cope with that, then welcome to the club!

4 The Defiant Ones
– the students' union explained

Andrew Garland

Now you've secured your place at university, you'll want to know more about that central pillar of student life, that guardian of all social and political activity – the students' union!

When registering for your course, you will be bombarded with information of all kinds regarding clubs, societies, parties, events, welfare, advice and many other services. A lot of that information will come from the university itself, and much will come from banks, local businesses and national companies who rely on the economic power of the student body. However, the majority of information that will be made available to you, and even forced upon you through leaflets, enthusiastic volunteers and displays of all kinds, will come from the students' union (SU).

At any welcome event laid on by the students' union, the various clubs and societies of the union will want you to know that they exist and will want your membership. In with them will be the students running the services designed to look after your welfare needs and those running voluntary services, such as community action groups. Whatever your interests in life, from rugby or canoeing to chess or drama, there is sure to be something for you on offer through the SU.

But for you as a student nurse, life at university will be very different from the other students. Your needs are often not fully understood by the university authorities, the SU or even nursing students themselves! The history of pre-registration nurse education in the university sector is short: degree level less than 20 years ago and diploma level just 10 years ago. Although there are some notable efforts at integration around the UK, the overall opinion is that students' unions have generally failed at providing services to and for the nursing student population. Indeed, it is still commonplace for nursing students to complete their three years without ever having collected their NUS cards.

Of course, this varies from place to place around the UK, but amazingly, the variation can also exist within an individual university from year to year. Academic and clinical commitments increase throughout the course, so the level of voluntary commitment an individual student may offer will become erratic. The later into the course the individual is, the less likely he or she will be willing or able to support any volunteer-based student activities beyond verbal approval.

Purpose of the students' union

All universities and higher education establishments have a union of students that exists to promote the interests and welfare of its membership and to respond to the general needs of its members. Membership is made up from the student population, and the membership creates and guides the structure and running of the union.

Regardless of the discipline being studied, all registered students of a university are entitled to membership of the SU. Therefore, all students should expect a service that reflects their needs, including addressing the concerns and views of the student population.

The university system

Although not widely publicised, membership of the students' union is entirely optional, and students can, on an individual basis, opt out of membership. However, many students are led to believe that they only become a part of the SU once they collect their membership card. But membership of a students' union is automatic following registration at the university (unless the relevant opt out paperwork is completed), with the National Union of Students membership card only being supplied to allow access to union facilities.

Should a student decide not to take up students' union membership (assuming he or she can find out how to do this), the university has an obligation to provide a similar standard of support as that provided by the students' union. Access to all services must be made possible so that no student is disadvantaged on the basis of membership.

The student services of the university should operate in cooperation with the students' union to avoid unnecessary duplication of work or services. However, some central services provided generally for students may not reflect the specific needs of particular student groups, so attention should be paid to ensuring faculty based services address specific needs. Naturally, this also applies to the SU.

The students' union and the National Union of Students

The students' union is the organisation of students that is attached to the individual establishment. The individual student is a member of the institution's SU. In contrast, the National Union of Students (NUS) comprises an affiliation of students' unions – in other words, it is the local SU that has membership of the NUS, not the individual student.

Students' union services

Each SU has a range of services that should be accessible to students. Many services are generic in nature, such as advisory services, and some are specifically targeted, such as for disabled students. Generally, students' unions will have facilities that provide food and drink. Some, depending on the size of the university, will have anything from discos to conference centres. All will have bars, but not necessarily on every campus. There will also be access to sports facilities.

The infrastructure of the union will depend on the size and number of buildings available, the size of the student population, the number of campuses to be catered for and the effectiveness of the strategies followed by the executive committee. Trading is important in generating revenue for the union and this effectively means that any profits generated through trading in this way can be put back into the union for the benefit of all students.

Welfare is an extremely important responsibility for an SU. In recent times, welfare services have had to respond to important issues such as HIV and

AIDS, meningitis, drug abuse, depression and hardship. To student nurses, much of what welfare does will sound like health promotion services, and that is exactly what many of them are, so it is worth being involved at this level.

They may provide:

- job search facilities;
- students' union run employment agencies;
- community action groups that work to build links to the local non-student communities;
- advisory services, including telephone helplines.

STRUCTURE OF A UNION

Students' unions are based around a written constitution that spells out the will of the membership in terms of the running and structure of the union. The constitution allows for a committee to exist that will take care of the day-to-day running of the union and will outline the powers at the disposal of that committee. The committee will consist of a number of students elected to specific posts for a one-year period. Of these elected posts, a number will allow for sabbatical officers, that is students who have taken a year out from their studies to give the role full time commitment. It is usually also possible for a student to take up a post immediately following graduation if he or she was elected while still a student. Usually, the elections take place during the second term of the academic year.

The constitution will make reference to policy documents that operate within the students' union, and these are detailed separately so that they can be altered and updated without changing the constitutional reference. All students of the union should have free access to the union constitution and all relevant policy documents.

GETTING INVOLVED

Involvement in the SU is possible and open to all registered students. However, having the right to be involved and being able to get involved is a completely different matter. The unions have always operated to serve the needs of the student population based on the usual academic year. With lengthy study weeks, clinical placements and all of the usual personal study and assignments to fit in, it is obvious that any involvement in the SU needs a tremendous effort on the part of student nurses. Even when this effort is made, maintaining involvement is not realistic without major changes to the structure of the union.

Executive meetings are usually weekly during traditional term times and are mostly open meetings, so any student can attend. In this setting, nursing students may feel intimidated by the authority of the executive committee, but this will almost certainly be due to the language barrier that exists. The structure of nurse education is massively complex in comparison to any other university course, and the language to describe the sets of rules, regulations and requirements that exist for nursing students to qualify and register can sound completely alien to the individual executive members.

Should you get little or no support from the SU executive, this is not the end of the line! Any students' union has a students' council in one form or another. This consists of the heads and chairs of various student committees and student representatives and has the role of ensuring that the executive always acts within the students' union constitution. Some students' councils have significant powers that can be used to overturn executive decisions, call emergency general meetings and even decide on interim policies to be put in place until a general meeting. Any approach to students' union executives should be backed with an approach to the students' council who will also hold regular open meetings.

General meetings are the ultimate arena in which to make effective changes to the students' union as they are the meetings of the membership. Such meetings should take place at least once per term. Decisions made at general meetings are binding and constitutional. The basic format follows an agenda which has to be set in advance of the meeting to a time deadline – for example, motions to go on the agenda must be submitted to the chair of the executive no later than 48 hours before the meeting. However, provision is made for emergency motions and details will be in the constitution. Such procedure is necessary to guard against sudden major decisions being made at meetings that may cause problems later on. Motions need to be well thought out and the arguments for and against the motion must be debated at the general meeting to give all parties fair input.

As a student nurse, any approaches to the students' union executive committee should result in discussion as to how services to nursing students can be improved. If constitutional changes need to be made to accommodate the needs of nursing students, the executive should support and assist in this happening as it is in its interests to help in the process of integration.

When making efforts to improve services from the students' union, student nurse representatives need to get faculty management on side. It is important to keep management informed of the efforts being made and the benefits that can be brought to the students of the faculty. If efforts have been made previously with any degree of success, new representatives will have an easier task in persuading management to support any initiatives. Why keep faculty so closely involved? Again, this is because of the nature of the course, and any flexibility in studies or clinical placements that can allow student representatives to attend meetings and events will need to be approved by faculty. It is possible to gain faculty support, and it can prove very effective, particularly when breaking new ground in union representation.

ADAPTING SERVICES TO NURSING STUDENTS

As mentioned, there is a difference between nursing students and the general student population. For degree students in nursing, the differences are less marked in terms of academic year, but for diploma students this is one of the major differences. Pre-registration diploma nursing is based on a timetable that is unrecognisable to most other students. Two intakes per year, with holiday schedules defined by cohort, means that diploma nursing students are either in the classroom or on clinical placements all year round. This does not fit in with the cycle of the academic year to which students' unions are accustomed, making it difficult for students of nursing to have services provided through the normal term or semester breaks.

For nurse education generally, the many differences are clear to nursing students, if not to the relevant authorities. The basic structure of the course, split into two 18-month periods with clinical placements averaging 50% of the time, is an immediate difference that has gone mostly unrecognised by those planning and implementing student services. Added to this is the longer time commitment to both lecture time and clinical time. The average hours committed to lectures for most university courses is 13 hours per week throughout term time. To attain registration as a qualified nurse, it is a requirement that a student completes 2,400 hours of classroom time and 2,400 hours of clinical time, and this works out to a 37.5 hour week. Immediately, it can be seen that it is difficult to define a nursing student as a student in the normal students' union sense.

Approaching the students' union president and discussing the situation for nursing students is a good first step, but should be backed up with attendance at executive meetings on a regular basis. There may be a history between previous nursing students and previous executive committees, and this is worth investigation to see what was achieved. It may be that the university provides nurse education across multiple sites and that one site has an active nursing student organisation. If this is so, the students' union executive should at least be aware that such activity exists and it can help you to make contact with such groups so that you can seek advice.

Nationally, there is plenty of help and support for nursing students who want to make a difference and get a better deal for themselves, their colleagues and future students. There are over 50,000 nursing students in the UK and the majority of them are members of the Royal College of Nursing (RCN). All pre-registration student members are automatically members of the Association of Nursing Students (ANS). The ANS is very well structured and organised to represent the views of the student membership of the profession, and has proven itself to be very effective over recent years in providing for the needs of nursing students.

The task for the ANS is vast, and it has long been realised that the national activities of the ANS executive must be backed by active student members locally. Student stewardship, branch meetings, regional and national student forums, along with workshops and seminars, ensure that the ANS has direct contact with its membership and the membership has ways in which to guide the executive.

The executive represents all four countries of the UK through nine elected student nurse representatives and a student adviser. Together, the executive committee guides the national activities of the student members and holds a student conference during September of each year. The professional conference, Congress, also plays host to many student members who are able to gain from the experience of debating student and professional issues. Issues such as clinical placements, mentorship, accommodation, attrition and harassment and bullying have been high on the agenda in recent times. The ANS has also led the way for the RCN in the joint union effort that created the 'Charter for Nursing and Midwifery Education' that has been adopted by many universities as a standard to apply to nurse education. Student members of the RCN who wish to find out more about local and national activities of the RCN/ANS and how to get involved can call RCN direct on 0345 726 100 for information. The ANS believes that improving services to nursing students from students' unions and university student services can help to reduce student attrition from nursing and give students a better experience of life as a student nurse. To this end, the RCN/ANS has a joint working agreement with the NUS and works hard at local levels with students' unions. As with the students' union, the input and participation of the ANS membership is critical when deciding on ways forward, and there is plenty of opportunity and support for those who wish to play an active part.

5 The Empire Strikes Back
– an explanation of the NHS

Eileen Walsh

The National Health Service, or NHS as it is more commonly known, celebrated its 50th anniversary on the 5th July 1998. It is one of the largest and most complex organisations operating in Britain. Many, if not all, of the population will at some time avail themselves of the services offered. As it is one of the largest employers in the public sector, it is important that all employees understand the complex structures that make up the NHS today.

During its lifetime, the NHS has witnessed a lot of organisational change. Some of these changes have been welcomed, while others have been greeted with scepticism and opposition. Nonetheless the NHS as it stands today has evolved with these changes and, as with all major organisations, has come to realise that change is an ongoing thing. However, in order to understand how the NHS works today, it is important to understand the history and origins of the organisation.

THE EARLY DAYS

From 1850 to 1900, doctors treated the upper and middle classes in their own homes, provided they could pay for this service. The hospitals of that time consisted of three main types: almshouses for the poor, infirmaries for contagious illnesses, such as tuberculosis, and asylums. The almshouses were voluntary hospitals that ran mainly on donations and tended to deal with short stay acute conditions. Public hospitals were workhouse type infirmaries that were locally controlled. As a result, they varied widely from region to region. The third type of hospital, the asylum, was set up for the protection of society from mental illness and the containment of antisocial conditions.

The net result of this system was that hospitals did not figure as a major provider of care as they tended to be places one went when there was nowhere else to go or there was no hope of getting better.

However, a number of factors impacted greatly on the organisation of healthcare provision. The first of these was the development of anaesthesia. The ability to successfully anaesthetise patients revolutionised the approach to surgical treatment as it meant that operations became safer and chances of survival were improved. As it was administered in hospitals, this caused a shift in perception of the role of hospitals. Now patients could be treated safely in hospital and then return home. Another event that contributed to change was the introduction of the 1858 Medical Act, which licensed only university-trained doctors to practise medicine. Prior to this act the profession was unlicensed and anyone could call themselves a doctor without necessarily having undergone accredited university training. In 1860, the Nightingale School of Nursing was established but unfortunately, unlike doctors, state registration for nurses was not introduced until 1919 – a situation which may have created the 'subordinate' position of nurses to doctors.

During this period, the state played a relatively active role in promoting better conditions for health, if not in the actual delivery of healthcare. It worked at developing better social conditions, such as sanitation and diet.

MOVING INTO THE 20TH CENTURY

The first half of the 20th century heralded more changes for the organisation of healthcare in Britain. Many were as a direct result of economic and social factors of that period. On a financial basis, hospitals struggled to match their income with the increasing costs of providing care. This resulted in voluntary hospitals grouping together to survive. Eventually, these hospitals were forced to introduce charging mechanisms to patients. In addition, in 1911, a form of voluntary health insurance was introduced, but it did not cover the population as a whole and was based on the ability to pay.

During the first part of the century, the role of the state became increasingly interventionist in its approach. Due to unemployment levels,

The Empire Strikes Back – an explanation of the NHS

it was forced to introduce welfare measures to appease the masses, and attempted to establish services at a minimum standard for the majority of the population. The government started to recognise health as its responsibility. It needed to ensure that the workforce remained healthy in order to support the economy, while at the same time there was a possible threat of world war.

In 1938, the Emergency Medical Service was formed. Due to the fear of mass casualties from a potential war, it was acknowledged that there was a need for greater coordination of hospital services, as well as national services for blood transfusion and ambulance services. In 1942, the publication of the Beveridge Report highlighted the duty of the state in relation to health and social security. Social conditions of the early 1940s and the impact of World War Two favoured the introduction of a more centralised approach by the government.

CREATING THE NHS

In post-war Britain, the Labour government wanted to create a national health service that was funded and owned by the state. This approach was a radical departure from the fragmented system of voluntary hospitals, and the pre-war system of voluntary health insurance. Despite a slower start than the social security scheme, the NHS came into being on 5th July 1948. It was founded on the basis of several underlying principles, which aimed to establish a health service that was accessible to the entire population. It would provide a full range of services, both preventative and curative, of the highest standards. Perhaps most importantly, this new NHS was to be free to all, at the point of delivery, financed from general taxation. Although these principles were welcomed by many, the British Medical Association was opposed to the proposed changes as it would affect the way in which it was organised and paid for.

The formation of the National Health Service in 1948 was a result of the National Health Service Act, which was passed in 1946. Health services were provided through hospital and primary care services with social services provided by local authorities. For the first time everyone could now register with a GP of their choice who could offer them free treatment. Any prescriptions for medicines prescribed by GPs could be filled free of charge at any pharmacy. If a GP could not treat any particular illness, he could refer the patient to a hospital consultant for more specialised treatment. Voluntary and public hospitals were nationalised under a single administrative system, which operated at two levels: Regional Hospital Boards and Hospital Management Committees. Services at these nationalised hospitals were free of charge, as were visits to opticians and dentists.

In order to administrate the hospital system, 14 Regional Hospital Boards were established. These Boards consisted of members, appointed by the Minister of Health, who were responsible for the overall organisation of the hospitals, deciding how many there should be, where they should be located and how they should be staffed. At a local level, each hospital had its own Hospital Management Committee appointed by the Regional Hospital Board. These committees were generally controlled by doctors who still retained control over who was admitted for treatment. The exceptions to this rule were the teaching hospitals, which remained governed by their own boards.

Over the next few years, support for the NHS grew and its popularity increased among the population. However, all was not well with the economy of that time and as pressures grew for tighter economic reforms, the NHS was also experiencing an increase in demand for its services. The costs for providing a national health service were greatly underestimated, as the projected uptake of services had been based on the level of demand that existed when patients had to pay. However, as the market barriers to entry into the system were removed, the demand grew rapidly.

ORGANISATIONAL CHANGES IN THE NHS

Over the past five decades, the NHS has seen three major restructures which have resulted in substantial changes to the way in which the management of the service is provided. The first of these changes came with what is commonly termed the 1974 NHS Reorganisation.

This reorganisation resulted in the Regional Hospital Boards and the Hospital Management Committees being replaced by 15 Regional Health Authorities (RHAs) and 90 Area Health Authorities (ARAs). The ARAs worked closely with Local Authorities and Family Practitioner Committees so as to promote coordination between the branches of health provision and to facilitate greater integration between health and social services. The overall style of management that this structure favoured was one of consensus management. It relied on team agreement in reaching decisions and these teams included doctors, nurses, administrators and finance personnel. In 1974, Community Health Councils were established to represent the views of the users of health services but this did not allow them to have input into any of the decisions regarding clinical services.

General changes in the economic climate, coupled with increased costs and increased demand, resulted in the introduction of cash limits on public expenditure for the NHS. This situation and the consensus style of management created little opportunity to develop planning for the NHS. Instead the system was seen as bureaucratic and inefficient.

In 1983, the Griffiths report proposed that the previous consensus style of management should be replaced by a system of general management throughout the NHS. These general managers would manage the NHS and would be judged on managerial performance against a variety of targets and indicators. Financial targets had to be met and managed. However, despite this responsibility, these general managers still did not have control over expenditure incurred by the clinical decisions made by the medical staff. As a result costs tended to be saved through cutting non-clinical services. Outside the hospital system, GPs continued to function free from the cash limits introduced previously for hospitals and operated as much clinical freedom as their funding would allow. Eventually, though, it became necessary to limit the type of drugs GPs prescribed due to rising costs.

Over the years the increased pressure for additional funding for the NHS necessitated another review of the NHS structure and resulted in the introduction of the concept of the internal market. The reforms led to the publication of a white paper entitled 'Working for Patients' which was published in 1989 and which formed the basis for the 1990 NHS and Community Care Act. These reforms created the purchaser/provider split in the NHS. Under this system the purchasing of healthcare was separated from the provision or delivery of healthcare. Health authorities and GPs would purchase healthcare on behalf of their resident populations from the hospitals and community services that provided them. Such purchasing decisions would be independent of the hospitals and other providers. GPs were given the option to become fundholding practices responsible for the direct purchase of certain services for their patients from their own discrete budgets. However, the reforms did not change the way that the NHS was funded and the method of funding through taxation continued.

The reforms were responsible for the creation of NHS trusts – hospitals and community services were allowed to become autonomous bodies who

Student survival guide

directly managed their own funds and services independent of the district health authorities. It was thought that this system would create open market competition with the introduction of the 'money following the patient' concept. It was believed that this concept would improve services resulting in greater accessibility, responsiveness and quality for the patient. On a strategic level, the NHS was re-organised to consist of a NHS Policy Board and a NHS Executive made up of eight regional offices.

This system of organisation has continued up to the present day with some changes, such as the mergers of Family Health Service Authorities with District Health Authorities, taking place along the way. In 1997, the government changed to a Labour administration and this resulted in the publication of new white papers on the NHS: The New NHS (England), Designed to Care (Scotland) and Putting Patients First (Wales). The changes proposed in these white papers came into being on 1st April 1999 and will have far reaching affects in the NHS. They involve some organisational change, with an emphasis on partnership, accountability, efficiency, quality standards and accessibility to services and information.

THE NHS IN ENGLAND

The NHS in England is made up of a number of different levels, ranging from the provider units up to parliament. The following section gives a brief synopsis of the main duties and functions of each group. It is not an exhaustive list of their extensive range of responsibilities.

Secretary of State

The NHS remains a state-funded system overseen by the Secretary of State for Health, supported by several ministers within the Department of Health. The Health Secretary is responsible to parliament for the provision of health services and can be questioned in parliament on any issues relating to the NHS, which acts as an accountability mechanism.

Department of Health

The Department of Health is responsible for the activities and workings of the entire NHS. It carries out a wide range of functions including setting the strategic framework for the NHS, securing and allocating resources and managing the overall performance and regulation of the NHS. In order to fulfil these functions the department is structured into three main divisions which interface with a number of other groups and agencies.

The responsibility for the development of NHS policy and strategic direction rests with the Department of Health. Guidance on priorities and planning is produced for cascading down the NHS structure on an annual basis to allow health authorities and trusts to plan for the services they need to purchase and deliver.

The Department of Health is responsible for securing resources for the NHS through the annual negotiation rounds of the public expenditure survey. Secured resources are subsequently allocated to the various health authorities across the country for further distribution on a local level.

One of the other major functions of the Department of Health is to monitor the performance of NHS organisations. In order to carry out this function, the department has developed the structure of the NHS Executive or NHSE. The NHSE deals with all operational issues involved in delivering the strategy passed down from the Department of Health.

NHS Executive

The NHSE consists of an executive board based at NHSE headquarters supported by eight regional offices. Each regional office is headed up by a regional director who is a member of the board. In addition each regional NHSE has a non-executive chairman who links closely with other chairmen to advise the Secretary of State on a variety of issues.

The NHS Executive plays an important role in linking the NHS to the government. It is mainly concerned with monitoring performance at a national level, developing and evaluating national policy and strategy and securing resources for allocation to health authorities, including managing capital allocations.

The eight regional NHS Executives support the overall NHSE system on a more local level. They are responsible for negotiating and agreeing contracts with the health authorities within their region. They monitor and review performance against these contracts in addition to monitoring individual trusts' performance in achieving statutory duties and in implementing national initiatives such as reducing waiting lists.

However, as with the NHSE headquarters, these offices perform a range of other functions to support the overall management of the NHS.

Health authorities

Prior to April 1996, health authorities were divided into two groups: District Health Authorities and Family Health Services Authorities. However, in 1996 these were merged into one type of organisation known simply as a Health Authority. These health authorities are managed by a board of members who consist of non-executive members and executive members. Executive members are full time employees, who manage both the operational and strategic aspects of the organisation, whereas non-executive members are appointed by the government to participate in the strategic management of the organisation.

Health authorities operate at a local level and they perform a range of functions for the population they serve. These can be broadly categorised into three main areas: strategy, support and monitoring. Within this range of functions, the authority is responsible for the purchase of healthcare provision on behalf of the local residents. Under the changes in the new white paper, health authorities will now take the lead in the development of the Health Improvement Programme. The purpose of this new programme is to develop a partnership approach to healthcare for a resident population by involving all the necessary groups responsible for health, social and environmental aspects. This programme should identify the needs of the local population and subsequently identify what needs to be done and by whom. The authority will be responsible for the purchase of health services to meet these needs. In addition to this purchasing role, the authority will continue to set and monitor local standards for services. Perhaps one of the biggest structural changes of this white paper is the abolition of GP fundholding, which will be replaced by Primary Care Groups. The authority will play a major supporting role in the development of these groups. The traditional role of the health authority will change significantly over the life of the changes proposed by the white paper. Eventually the authority will withdraw from the purchasing of healthcare and will adopt more of a monitoring and communication role.

NHS trusts: acute, community and mental health provider units

The introduction of the NHS reforms in the early 1990s brought with it the establishment of a new type of organisation called NHS trusts. Under previous structures, hospital and community services provided healthcare under the direct control of the District Health Authority and were referred to as directly managed units. With the introduction of the purchaser/provider split, the opportunity arose to allow these hospitals to become independent of the health authorities and to be responsible for organising and managing their own affairs in relation to the delivery of healthcare. Each trust has its own board of directors who are responsible for the performance of the trust, which, in turn, is monitored by the NHS Executive regional offices. Performance is monitored on a regular basis and all trusts have certain statutory duties to meet. Each trust is responsible for negotiating contracts with its purchasers to provide healthcare for its resident population.

As with health authorities, trusts will start to experience the white paper changes in the near future. Trusts will be required to adopt a collaborative partnership approach in line with the development of health improvement programmes. There will be a requirement for trusts to make information on services and costs readily available. Trusts will be required to place a renewed emphasis on quality standards, efficiency and effectiveness.

Primary Care Groups

The early 1990s also saw the introduction of structural changes for GPs throughout the UK. With the advent of the purchaser/provider split the opportunity arose to allow GPs to manage certain aspects of purchasing healthcare for their own patients. This concept was referred to as fundholding. Under the new white paper, this concept has been abolished completely and has been replaced by Primary Care Groups (PCGs). A PCG will typically contain a number of GP practices across a locally agreed and defined area. These groups will consist of GPs and their nursing services operating as a cohesive group within that area. It is hoped that by working in partnership with providers and other relevant groups the PCGs can purchase and monitor services for their populations while achieving better integration and access across primary and secondary boundaries. Initially, PCGs will be accountable to their health authority and their performance will be monitored by the authority. The introduction of PCGs will be a phased development with a spectrum of responsibility available to each PCG, dependent on ability and appropriateness as assessed by the health authority. It is envisaged that with time, PCGs will develop to trust status.

Special health authorities

Some healthcare services are managed on a national as opposed to a local level. In order to ensure that a national strategic and operational perspective is maintained these services are managed by special health authorities.

Community health councils

These councils were established to represent the interests and viewpoints of the public on healthcare issues and services. The members of the councils are voluntary with the exception of the chief officer and administrative staff who are employed to support the council.

VARIATIONS ON THE NHS ACROSS THE UK

Scotland

Until April 1999, the NHS in Scotland was the responsibility of the Secretary of State for Scotland supported by the Home and Health Department of Scotland. With devolution, this responsibility has passed to the new Scottish parliament. Changes under the new Scottish white paper have retained the purchaser/provider split of the old regime but have abolished the concept of the internal market and GP fundholding. The overall management of the NHS is carried out by a management executive that is responsible for policy, strategy and performance management. Fifteen health boards carry out the local strategy and monitoring functions. These boards previously performed purchasing and planning functions at a hospital level and also managed the primary care services for their resident populations. Under the new proposals, the health boards will continue to commission services from NHS trusts as defined by their Health Improvement Programme. As in England, all trusts will be expected to fully participate in the partnership approach to the development of a Health Improvement Programme. The difference between England and Scotland lies in the fact that the changes propose only two types of trust for Scotland in the future: acute trusts and Primary Care Trusts (PCTs). Unlike in England, it is proposed that these PCTs operate at full trust status with responsibility for the planning, purchasing and provision of all primary care services for their resident populations. In addition, it is planned to reduce the number of acute trusts.

As with the NHS in England, 'national' services such as the ambulance and blood transfusion services are organised by a common services agency. The NHS in Scotland also has 18 local health councils who represent the views of patients and public.

Wales

Until 1999, the NHS in Wales was the direct responsibility of the Secretary of State for Wales, based at the Welsh Office. With the establishment of the Welsh Assembly, this responsibility will transfer to the assembly and will probably be administered via the Welsh Health Department. The NHS in Wales currently has five health authorities that report directly into the Welsh Office as there are no regional NHSE offices in Wales. During the past year the number of acute and community trusts in Wales has been radically reduced through a series of mergers which resulted in combined acute and community trusts. These trusts relate to health authorities in a similar way to their English counterparts and will be expected to participate in the partnership approach to the development of local Health Improvement Programmes. All trusts will be subject to the growing emphasis on quality as a statutory duty. GP fundholding has been abolished in Wales and has been replaced with Local Health Groups (LHGs) which are similar in concept to PCGs but will operate as sub-committees of health authorities. The LHGs will be responsible for the purchasing of primary care services and, as time progresses, will assume budgetary responsibility evolving towards the PCT model.

Northern Ireland

The system in Northern Ireland operates slightly differently to its counterparts in the rest of the United Kingdom. At present it consists of an integrated approach to planning and provision of health and social services for the resident population. Similar to the former Welsh system, the responsibility for this service rests with the Secretary of State via the Northern Ireland Department of Health and Social Services and Management Executive. This department is supported by four integrated health and personal social services boards who oversee the planning and commissioning of all health and social services for their resident populations. Services are approved by 19 health and social services trusts, with GP services provided on a fundholding basis until 31st March 1999. In preparation for the end of fundholding, five GP commissioning groups have been introduced on a pilot scheme basis.

FEEDING THE BEAST: FUNDING THE NHS

Funding the NHS is a constant source of debate and is of great interest to the general public as a subject very dear to the nation's heart. However, it is important to understand the basic funding structure to appreciate the limits within which the current NHS operates and how it is important to manage the public's expectations of what the NHS can provide. There are various formulae and mechanisms by which the funding is calculated and distributed down the system, the complexity of which do not allow it to be explored in this text.

However, by way of a basic explanation of the financing system, the NHS is funded primarily through taxation. This means that the NHS competes with other government departments for a share of the public purse. All departments put forward their proposals and projected financial requirements for the budgetary period. There are no fixed or definite levels of funding guaranteed for the NHS and all funding requests compete for one pot of money. The division of resources can be influenced by several factors at any time but generally tends to be based on what is happening on economic, social and, more importantly, political fronts.

Once the overall allocation has been decided for the Department of Health a system of cascading down begins. The eight regional NHS Executives compete for their share of the pot on the basis of the needs of their areas and a range of other issues, such as future developments, service improvements and changing demography. At this point funding for national services such as the National Blood Transfusion service is topsliced out of the allocation. The regional NHS Executives are then responsible for distributing the resources down to the next level, the health authorities. At the next level down, health authorities distribute the resources amongst the providers: the NHS trusts, other specialist providers, previously GP fundholders and in future PCGs. However, it is worth noting that resources can also leak out of the NHS funding cycle when they are allocated for the purchase of services provided by private sector units. Examples of this are found in the provision of mobile MRI scanners by the technology companies. In most cases it is more cost effective for an organisation to buy in a highly technologically driven service instead of having to constantly invest capital in keeping up with the pace of change in technological advances.

This very basic explanation makes no attempt to deal with the various intricacies of NHS finance, such as external financing limits, capital charges or private finance initiatives.

WHAT LIES AHEAD?

The end of the millennium heralds yet another era of change for the NHS in the United Kingdom. In its 50 years of existence it has been no stranger to change – some good, some bad. The future holds some good ideas and fine aspirations for the NHS, such as the Commission for Health Improvement, which will support and oversee the concept of clinical governance and accountability. The changes will also see the introduction of the National Institute of Clinical Excellence, which aspires to promote clinical and cost-effective practice through the establishment of guidelines and the introduction of National Service Frameworks.

A new approach to partnership and collaborative working is being heralded as the way forward for adopting a more holistic approach to healthcare through the development of Health Improvement Programmes and Health Action Zones. Perhaps this approach will indeed be the light at the end of the tunnel for greater integration between all aspects of health, social services, environmental planning, education and so on. But who knows – although there is light, sometimes it can be a very long tunnel.

6 The Matrix – glossary of terms and anatomical positions

Phillip Hufton

As students beginning a nursing course, you will be bombarded by all manner of bewildering terms and words that will both amaze and confuse you.

Like any profession, healthcare has its own language and, though a concerted effort is made in most quarters not to use jargon, it is inevitable that you will come across it in your everyday life. Jargon aside, medical terms are another form of language that will not be familiar to most of you. Some of these seemingly complicated words and terms may be daunting to you at first. However, they can be broken down easily into a more digestible and understandable form. This chapter is by no means exhaustive, but acts merely as a guide. You will probably find it useful to supplement this information with a good nurse's dictionary, available from most good bookshops, for example The Oxford Concise Dictionary of Nursing or Bailière's Nursing Dictionary.

MEDICAL TERMINOLOGY

Most medical terminology is derived from early Greek or Latin words for example:

- *Card* (heart)
- *Haem* (blood)
- *Pneumon* (lung)

Unfortunately, many medical terms were developed at a time when the working of the human body was only partially understood, so in some

The Matrix – glossary of terms and anatomical positions

cases the terminology no longer appears appropriate. For example, hydrocephalus literally means water on the head, but the condition is caused by an accumulation of cerebrospinal fluid within the cranial vault. So although the name is inaccurate it continues to be used.

Medical terms are made up of a root with a combining vowel, usually an 'o', plus prefixes and suffixes that alter or modify the meaning of the root. For example:

Heam	–	*o*	–	*poiesis*
This is the root meaning blood		This is the combining vowel		This is the suffix meaning production, or formation of

Haemopoiesis, therefore, means production or formation of blood cells.

What follows are some examples of the more commonly used roots and their meanings. Hopefully these will help you understand and identify some of the conditions, and the terms used to describe them, that you will encounter during your training.

ROOTS

Roots are basic medical words.

Root	Meaning
A	
Abdomin/o	Abdomen
Ambly/o	Dull or dim
Angi/o	Vessel (usually a blood vessel)
Arteri/o	Arterial
Arthr/o	Joint
B	
Brachi/o	Arm
Bronchi/o	Bronchus
C	
Capit/o	Head
Cardi/o	Heart
Cephal/o	Head
Cervic/o	Neck, neck of the womb

Student survival guide

Root	Meaning
Cerebell/o	Cerebellum of the brain
Cholangi/o	Common bile duct
Col/o	Colon
Colp/o	Vagina
Cry/o	Cold
Crypt/o	Hidden
Cyst/i/o	Bladder, cyst or sac
Cyt/o	Cell
E	
Encephal/o	Brain
Enter/o	Intestines
F	
Faci/o	Face
G	
Gastr/o	Stomach
H	
Hepat/ico/o	Liver
Hist/o	Tissue
Hyster/o	Uterus
I	
Ile/o	Ileum
Isch/o	Deficiency blockage
K	
Kin/e/o	Movement/motion
L	
Lymph/o	Lymphatic vessels or lymphocytes
M	
Mast/o	Breast
Mening/o/i	Membranes covering brain and spinal cord
Myel/o	Bone marrow or spinal cord
Myring/o	Ear drum
Mal-	Bad
Meat/o	Opening
Meg/a/alo/aly	Large, oversized
Morph/o	Form, shape, structure
Myc/o	Fungus

The Matrix – glossary of terms and anatomical positions

Root	Meaning
N	
Necr/o	Death
Nephr/o	Kidney
Neur/o	Nerve
O	
Occipit/o	Back of the head
Oophor/o	Ovary
Opthalm/o	Eye or eyes
Orchi/o/do	Testes
Orth/o	Straight, normal, correct
Oss/eo/i and ost/e/eo	Bone or bones
P	
Pachy/o	Thick
Phleb/o	Vein or veins
Pneum/o/a	Lungs or respiration
Proct/o	Rectum or anus
Pulm/o	Lungs
Pyel/o	Pelvis or kidney
R	
Rhin/o	Nose
Rachi/o	Spine
Rect/o	Rectum
Ren/i/o	Kidney
S	
Splen/o	Spleen
Spondyl/o	Vertebrae or spinal cord
T	
Thorac/o	Chest
Tend/o	Tendon
Thyr/o	Thyroid gland
U	
Ureter/o	Ureter
Urethr/o	Urethra
V	
Vas/o	Vessel or duct
Ven /e /i/ o	Vein or veins

Table 6.1 Roots and their meanings

SUFFIXES

A suffix is the end of the word, the part of the word that follows the word root and adds to or modifies its meaning.

Suffix	Meaning	Example
-algia	a painful condition	neuralgia – pain that affects nerves
-ary	connected with	ovary – connected with the ovum
-ate	action or state	degenerate – to decline in condition
-cle, -culum, -cule	diminutive	molecule – small physical unit
-ectasia, -ectasis	a dilated or distended state	bronchiectasis – dilation of the bronchi
-ectomy	cutting out	appendectomy – cutting out of the appendix
-ia	state, condition	septicaemia – poisoning of the blood
-ic	pertaining to	manic – affected with madness
-ile	characteristic of	febrile – characteristic of fever
-ion	process, action	flexion – act of bending
-ism	condition, state	rheumatism – inflammation of muscles and joints
-itis	inflammation	appendicitis – inflammation of the appendix
-logy	body of knowledge	biology – knowledge of living organisms
-lysis	disintegration, dissolution	haemolysis – dissolution of red cells
-paenia	deficiency	thrombocytopaenia – deficiency of thrombocytes (platelets)
-plegia	paralysed state	hemiplegia – paralysis of one side of the body

The Matrix – glossary of terms and anatomical positions

Suffix	Meaning	Example
-poiesis	formation, production of	haemopoiesis – formation of red cells
-rrhagia	fluid discharge	lymphorrhagia – a flow of lymph
-rrhaphy	a suturing in place	gastrorrhaphy – surgical suture of the stomach
-rrhoea	flow	diarrhoea – frequent intestinal evacuations
-tomy	cut into, incision	tracheotomy – cutting into the trachea
-sis	state or process	haematemesis – vomiting blood

Table 6.2 Suffixes and their meanings

ANATOMICAL POSITION

Anatomical position is a reference system, used to locate parts and areas of the human body. In defining anatomical position, imagine that the patient is facing you, standing upright, arms loosely at sides, palms of the hands facing forward, head erect, eyes looking forward.

Right and left sides refer to the *patient's* right and left sides, *not yours*.

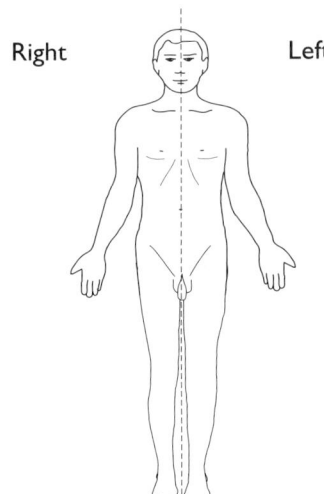

Fig 6.1

Student survival guide

The **median line** is an imaginary line drawn down the middle of the body (see Fig 6.2). Parts of the body nearest the median line are described as **medial** and those further away are referred to as **lateral**. For example, the cartilages of the knee joint are described as the medial and lateral meniscus.

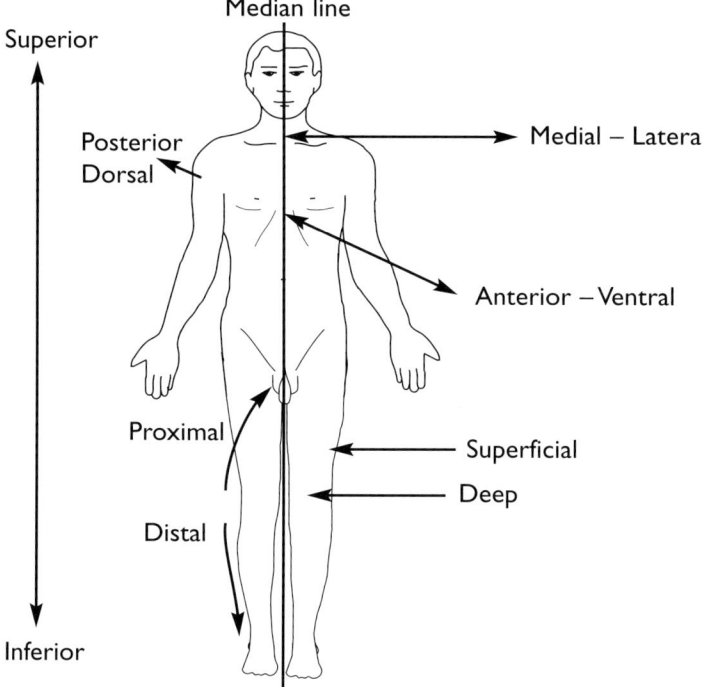

Fig 6.2

Superior	Towards the head, upper
Inferior	Away from the head, lower
Anterior	Ventral, front
Posterior	Dorsal, back
Proximal	Nearest to point of origin or attachment
Distal	Furthest from point of origin or attachment
Superficial	Near the surface of the body
Deep	Away from the surface of the body

The Matrix – glossary of terms and anatomical positions

The regions of the head and trunk can be divided into cephalic, thoracic, abdominal and pelvic.

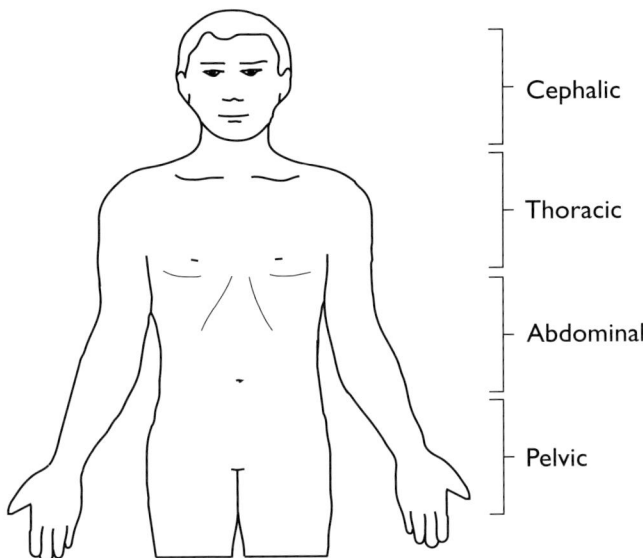

Fig 6.3

The abdominopelvic regions are divided into four quarters or quadrants.

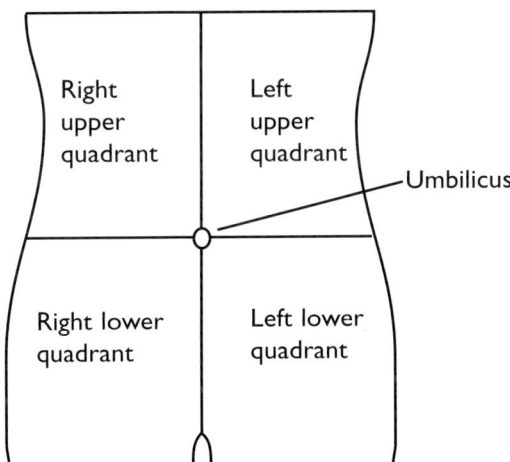

Fig 6.4

Student survival guide

Alternatively the abdominopelvic region can be divided into nine regions (see Fig 6.5). This can be useful in describing the position of pelvic pain.

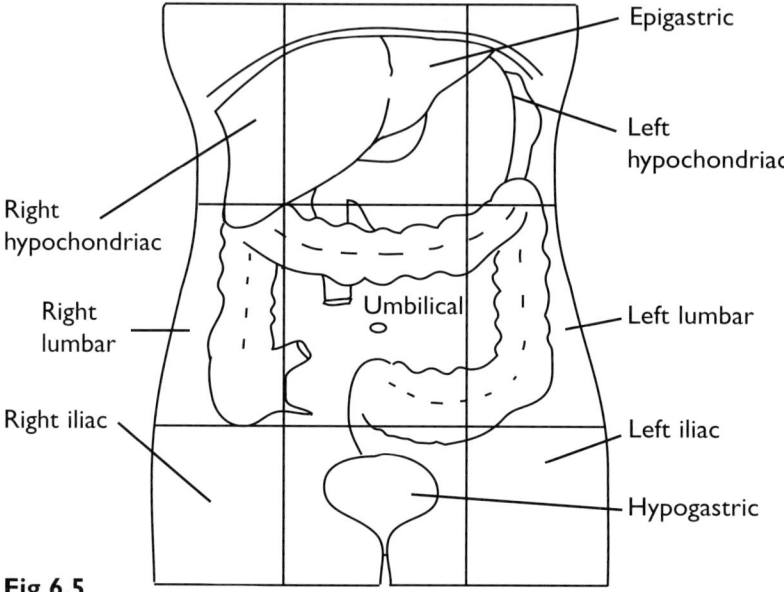

Fig 6.5

ABBREVIATIONS

What follows is a short list of some of the more common abbreviations that you may come across during your training. You will find these written in care plans, medical reports and so on. This list is by no means exhaustive, and you will no doubt be able to add to it as time goes by.

A
abd	abdomen
ADD	attention deficit disorder
ADH	anti-diuretic hormone
ALs	activities of living
AFP	alpha-foetoprotein
ASD	atrial-septal defect

B
BMR	basal metabolic rate
BPH	benign prostatic hypertrophy

The Matrix – glossary of terms and anatomical positions

Bpm	beats per minute
BSE	breast self examination

C
CAD	coronary artery disease
C&S	culture and sensitivity
Cath	catheter
CCU	coronary care unit
CF	cystic fibrosis
CMV	cytomegalovirus
CPAP	continuous positive airway pressure
CVP	central venous pressure
CVS	chorionic villi sampling

D
D&V	diarrhoea and vomiting
DNA	did not attend
DNA	deoxyribonucleic acid
DRG	diagnosis related groups

E
ECMO	extracorporeal membrane oxygenation
EDD	estimated date of delivery

F
FBS	fasting blood sugar
FHR	foetal heart rate
FSH	follicle stimulating hormone

H
HBV	Hepatitis B virus
Hib	Haemophilus influenzae type b
HIV	Human Immunodeficiency Virus

I
ICP	intracranial pressure
ICS	intercostal space
ICU	Intensive Care Unit
IQ	intelligence quotient

J
JRA	juvenile rheumatoid arthritis

L
LBW	low birth weight

LMP	last menstrual period	
LOC	level/loss of consciousness	

M
MMR	measles mumps and rubella	

N
N/A	not applicable	
NBM	nil by mouth	
NSAID	non-steroidal anti-inflammatory drug	
NSR	normal sinus rhythm	

O
OPD	out patient department	
OT	occupational therapy	

P
PCA	patient controlled anaesthetic	
PID	pelvic inflammatory disease	
PRN	as required	
PUO	pyrexia of unknown origin	
Px	pneumothorax	

R
RA	rheumatoid arthritis	
RNA	ribonucleic acid	
RDS	respiratory distress syndrome	

S
SIDS	sudden infant death syndrome	
SLE	systemic lupus erythematosus	

T
TCI	to come in	
TTH	to take home	
TPN	total parental nutrition	
TSE	testicular self examination	
Tx	treatment	

7 Other People's Money
– managing your finances

Zosia Kmietowicz

WHAT IS A BURSARY?

All students who take a degree or diploma course in nursing or midwifery are eligible for a NHS bursary. A bursary is a grant or allowance to cover day-to-day living costs while studying.

Students on diploma courses all receive a flat rate basic maintenance grant. It is not means-tested and no contribution is required from a student's own income or from his or her family.

Students who take a degree in nursing or midwifery are treated like all other degree students and their bursaries are means-tested. This means that your own income, and that of your parents or spouse, will be taken into account when your bursary is awarded. The amount of grant you receive will depend on this income and your parents or spouse are expected to make up the amount that is deducted.

HOW MUCH IS A BURSARY?

Nursing students taking a degree are awarded a basic NHS bursary of £2,225 if they are studying in London, £1,180 for studying elsewhere, and £1,480 if they are living at home. This amount can be topped up to £5,200

Student survival guide

with extra allowances or a student loan for those on full-time courses (see Table 7.1).

The basic bursary for full-time student nurses taking a diploma is £5,374 for students in London and £4,572 for those outside London or living at home. With extra allowances this amount can be topped up to £6,000 (see Table 7.1).

Extra allowances

There are a number of extra allowances available to nursing students that may be added to the basic bursary for those eligible.

Allowance	Degree students	Diploma students
Extra weeks' attendance	Available for courses longer than 30 weeks and 3 days.	Available to those who have to move to London for placement.
Older students' allowance	Available to those over 26.	Available to those over 26.
Dependants' allowances	Available for spouse and children.	Available for spouse and children.
Single parent addition	Available	N/A
Two homes grant	Available	N/A
Excess travel expenses	Available for placements.	Available for placements.
Disabled students' allowances	Available	N/A
Student loans	Available	N/A
Access funds and hardship loans	Available	N/A
NHS hardship grant	Available	N/A

Table 7.1 Extra allowances for degree and diploma students

These extra allowances can make a big difference to the amount of total bursary you receive so it is important to provide all relevant information

Other People's Money – managing your finances

in your bursary application. For example, the single parent addition currently runs at £1,000 over 52 weeks for single students with a child or children (it cannot, however, be paid in addition to the older students' allowance). Students with dependants can also be awarded an extra £425 to £2,025 depending on the people who are financially dependent on them – children or a spouse.

Tuition fees

Student nurses on diploma or degree courses do not have to pay tuition fees. These are paid for by the Department of Health.

Receiving payment

When you have been accepted on either a nursing degree or diploma course you will be sent an application form for a bursary by the NHS Student Grants Unit (SGU). Once this has been filled in the amount of bursary you are entitled to will be worked out and you will be notified of your award. All special circumstances, such as dependants, anticipated travel and so on, will be taken into account when your bursary is calculated. Payments will normally be made monthly in advance, the first by cheque and then by credit transfer. You should therefore try to make sure you have opened a bank account before your course starts. Any excess travel expenses are normally made each quarter in arrears and added to the next instalment.

EXTRA FINANCIAL ASSISTANCE

Student loans

Nursing students on degree courses may be entitled to a student loan to cover the balance of living costs (those on part time courses or on postgraduate level courses are not). Bursaries are not meant to meet all your maintenance costs, so it is worth considering taking out a loan to avoid hardship while you are studying.

Loans are available via your local education authority (LEA) and you should apply for one before your course starts. The LEA will inform the Student Loans Company of the maximum loan you are entitled to. It is then up to you to decide how much of the loan, if any, you want from the Student Loans Company. Your LEA will be able to give you more advice.

The way you will have to repay your loan is worked out on the basis of your income after you graduate. You only start repaying your loan when your income is above the income threshold, which is set at £10,000 a year for those starting to repay in the year 2000. The amount you repay is based on a percentage of your income. For example, if you are earning £12,000 you will be required to repay £3 a week. Repayments are generally collected by the Inland Revenue from the start of the tax year (April 6) after you have finished your course. If your income ever falls below the threshold level, your repayments are suspended. If a graduate's income remains less than £10,000 throughout his or her working life, no repayments will be needed.

Access funds and hardship loans

If you are still finding it hard to manage on a bursary and loan, extra money is available in the way of funds and hardship loans. Your college or students' union will be able to give you more information. Again, only students on degree courses are eligible.

NHS hardship grant

In exceptional circumstances students on means-tested bursaries may be eligible for a NHS hardship grant. You must have taken up your full loan entitlement to apply. Ask your college for more information.

Council Tax and benefits

All full time students, including those on diploma courses, are either exempt from Council Tax or are entitled to discounts. In certain circumstances you may be eligible for Council Tax Benefit, Housing Benefit and social security benefits. For advice about all benefits you should contact your local authority or Benefits Agency office.

BOOSTING YOUR BURSARY

However much your bursary adds up to many student nurses find it is just not enough to cover their living expenses and look to boost their income by taking on some kind of work. You can earn up to your personal allowance (£4,433 for the 1999/2000 tax year) without paying tax although you will have to pay National Insurance if you earn more than £64 a week.

It is more difficult for student nurses to find work than other students because of the hours and shift work involved in nurse training. (Student nurses generally study for 45 weeks of the year as opposed to 30 weeks for ordinary degree course students.) Students on degree courses are more flexible and may want to consider taking a part time evening job in a pub or restaurant, for example, or working for the Post Office during the Christmas holidays. Diploma course students are more restricted, but many find work as care assistants through nurse banking agencies, which helps build up experience in nursing while still studying. Contact the student job shop in your students' union or look up nursing agencies in your local Yellow Pages for more information.

Another option is taking a gap year before starting college to save up some money while working full time so that you have a pool of cash when you take up your course.

BUDGETING

Learning to manage your money can be the most difficult aspect of student life. But taking the time to think about what money you have and the expenses you are going to encounter during your student years is time well spent. It can stop you getting into debt and mounting up bills which can take time and effort to sort out – time that is probably better spent on doing course work or earning some money from a part time job.

To take control of your spending the first thing you need to do is to work out how much money you need to survive. Add up all your expenses, such as rent, travel, food, bills, uniforms and stationery, to give you an idea of what you will need to pay for. A budget has to be accurate to be effective, so try to think of everything you might need. It is also important to be absolutely honest. For example if you like to go out, budget for it and try to be realistic about how much you spend on beer or wine.

Once you know the amount of the bursary you will be awarded you can compare your income with your expected expenditure. If these figures do not tally or your expenses far outweigh your bursary you will have to think of ways of increasing your income or cutting your out-goings. Once you have worked out a reasonable budget where you do not end up overdrawn a month after starting your course, try to stick to your plans. Follow your spending guide as closely as possible and try to avoid impulse spending. It is important to review your budget from time to time to make sure you are not overspending. When you take money out of the bank you usually get a balance. Make sure this matches what you think you should have in the bank and if it doesn't find out where the money has gone and adjust your spending accordingly.

How to survive – basic dos and don'ts when living on a low income

Do

- sort out your bursary and other entitlements quickly;
- make sure you know how the system works if you are taking out a student loan;
- budget carefully, even before starting your course;
- keep a record of what you spend and where you spend it;
- take advantage of free banking facilities for students and free overdrafts if you need one;
- open all letters from your bank when you get them and reply to them promptly;
- acknowledge that if you get into debt it can affect you emotionally and seriously distract you from your studies;
- seek advice as soon as things start to get out of control – the longer you leave a problem the harder it will be to sort out;
- allow some money for going out and enjoying yourself.

Don't

- overspend at the beginning of your first term – remember your money has to last you all year;
- buy non-essentials when you are struggling to pay for basics;
- ignore signs that spending is getting out of control;
- guess at what you are spending;
- be afraid to ask for advice if you are having financial problems;
- cut yourself off from family and friends;
- make rash promises to pay when you know you can't;
- exceed your overdraft limit without first asking for authorisation – unauthorised overdraft rates are very high when compared with what is offered if you stick within agreed limits;
- get paranoid! Remember you will not be student forever and your bank or building society will see you as a good long-term investment, so approach them with confidence.

MAKING YOUR MONEY GO FURTHER

Here are some practical tips on surviving the student years.

- Live near to where you will spend most of your student time to minimise travel costs.
- Look for cheap accommodation. Halls of residence are a good option, but if not available look for cheap alternatives, such as housing associations and shared houses.
- Make the most of student nurse discounts. You can save money on many things such as travel, cinema visits, haircuts, exhibitions, concerts and so on.
- Avoid expensive habits such as casinos and nightclubs.
- Try to restrict nights out to the weekend as going out every night can make a big hole in your budget.

Student survival guide

- Shop around. Buy second hand textbooks if possible (from students in the year above you or from the students' union) or use the library. Try second hand clothes shops if you want something new.
- Long hospital shifts may mean you need to buy a number of meals each day at the canteen. Take sandwiches for at least one meal to avoid spending too much.
- Try to buy economy value brands at supermarkets.
- If living in a shared house try to shop for food with friends – buying in bulk can save money.

USEFUL CONTACTS

If you have any enquires about financial support contact the following agencies, depending on where you plan to study.

England

The NHS Student Grants Unit

Room 212c Government Buildings

Norcross

Blackpool FY5 3TA

Tel: 01253 856123

Scotland

The Student Awards Agency for Scotland

3 Redheughs Rigg

South Gyle

Edinburgh EH12 9HH

Tel: 0131 556 8400

Wales

The Welsh Health Common Services Agency

Education Purchasing Unit
Ground Floor CP2
Welsh Office Cathays Park
Cardiff CF1 3NQ
Tel: 029 2082 5111

Northern Ireland

Department of Education for Northern Ireland

Rathgael House
Balloo Road
Bangor, Co Down
BT19 7PR
Tel: 01247 279418

OTHER USEFUL ADDRESSES

Student Loans Company Ltd

100 Bothwell Street
Glasgow G2 7JD
Tel: 0800 405 0101
Fax: 0141 306 2005

English National Board for Nursing, Midwifery and Health Visiting

Victory House
170 Tottenham Court Road
London W1P 0HA
Tel: 020 7388 3131
Fax: 020 7383 4031
Email: enb.careers@easynet.co.uk

Student survival guide

UCAS

Fulton House
Jessop Avenue
Cheltenham
Gloucestershire GL50 3SH
Tel: 01242 227788
Fax: 01242 221622

Nursing and Midwifery Admissions Service

Fulton House
Jessop Avenue
Cheltenham
Gloucestershire GL50 3SH
Tel: 01242 544949
Fax: 01242 263555

8 Payback – where to find help and support

Andrew Garland

STARTING OUT

Embarking on a course of study in nursing takes well planned, advanced preparation, meaning that help must be available before commencing the course. Without that help, many students would not be able to organise their lives sufficiently in advance of the given start date. Issues such as childcare, transport and accommodation must be resolved so that an individual student can begin this new life with the minimum of fuss. Accurate information is essential to the prospective student so that he or she may feel secure in making the decision to begin an intensive course of study.

Currently, the systems in place to facilitate such organisation are patchy and without any national guidelines. More surprisingly, the help, advice and other welfare available to nursing students throughout the course leave a lot to be desired. The need for assistance at all levels, financial, professional and counselling support amongst many, is obvious throughout the course, but it is the nature of the course that can make many essential services inaccessible for most nursing students.

Often, the fact that nursing students can find it difficult to access services translates to lack of demand for those very services. This can be used as justification to cut existing services or to not establish them in the first place.

However, nursing is still a sought after course of study throughout most of the UK, so what help is available to students from initial inquiry through to qualification? And how can welfare be better directed to suit the needs of this most unique and diverse group of students?

Advice available

Approaching the institution where you would like to study is a starting point. Most have recruitment days at which information is available about the demands of the course and how it is likely to affect lifestyle. Sometimes, the recruitment drive can be in the form of a 'road show' which can give students the opportunity to get the necessary information at a local venue. This is particularly useful for those interested in nursing that may live in areas some distance from the institution.

Nurse lecturers will staff any such event across all disciplines being offered, so an individual can be directed to the information and literature of most relevance. If a prospective student is unsure about the structure of the course and the career paths available, recruitment events are the place to get the information regarding all disciplines (adult, mental health, learning disabilities and child branches) and how the course approaches them.

Remember, though, that a recruitment event for an institution has the aim of attracting students to study at a particular university and, as such, there may be some pressure applied for application forms to be completed at the event. This tactic works well when an institution has a 'direct entry' programme, meaning that the prospective student may not have to go through a clearing system (UCAS or NMAS), but caution should be exercised, particularly if there has been no contact with any other institution.

Careers advice centres may have information available on the course of study, although many would-be nursing students have found this to be lacking in content or accuracy at times. This will depend where the advice centre is located and how much demand they have had for information about pre-registration nursing. Also, the advice given needs to come from someone who has knowledge and awareness of the pre-registration nursing education system. After all, this is a highly complex system, subjected to many rapid changes, and there are variations across the UK in the implementation of the academic and clinical practice components.

Well presented information and advice from a knowledgeable careers adviser, cross referenced with the information provided by an institution, is a fairly good way to assess the suitability of the course for the individual.

Talking to nursing students can be helpful. This can give new students a positive feel of nursing and avoid some of the negativity that those who are disillusioned can portray. Those involved locally in students' union activities will have a clear picture about what is available to nursing students and what work is being done to make facilities and services more readily available at their institution.

The Royal College of Nursing has a network of student activists taken from the student membership. They are well organised, with good resources and have the intention of improving the situation in pre-registration nurse education. They are often the first points of contact for student members seeking advice and support and, as such, it is important that student stewards have access to information and support systems that can deliver that support.

WHO CAN HELP?

Careers officers, nurse tutors, staff nurses and existing nursing students can all give relevant information regarding life as a student nurse. It is a good idea for prospective students to talk with a range of people so that a broader picture can be built before making a final decision. However, many of us have a preconceived or media image of nursing and the education that is provided. This allows many to believe that they have all of the necessary information that can lead them to the correct decision in their choice of course and, for some, this can cause problems that may seem insurmountable at the time.

WHO SHOULD HELP?

All of the people mentioned in the previous paragraph should be helpful to students or prospective students. Careers office staff are employed to provide up to date information on courses of study available, but this should not be relied on. The most up to date material will be available from a few other sources. These include the RCN, local institutions, the

National Boards for Nursing and Midwifery and the UKCC. Most of this information can also be accessed via the relevant websites.

WHAT CAN BE IMPROVED?

Systems of welfare specific to nursing and midwifery students are needed in the education system of today. This may seem obvious to those student activists and tutors/managers within the system, but is not so obvious to the fundholders and welfare providers concerned. It takes relevant evidence to make the necessary and much needed changes to the system as it exists so that services are better targeted to the needs of nursing students.

However, changes are being made in all areas and this is constantly improving the services available, particularly for new and prospective nursing students. As problems are highlighted, organised student activists are increasingly taking a proactive approach to seeking solutions. Often, it is evidence that is needed to support the drive for change and organised student groups can provide the opportunities for such evidence to be collected, be it anecdotal, written or in data form.

To illustrate, students at the University of North Wales, Bangor had many long-term concerns regarding the input and support of the students' union. A variety of approaches to dealing with this problem were explored and tried, but often the effect was short-term with the same barriers to progress appearing on a yearly cycle.

The main barrier was identified as a communication problem that crossed all levels. The cyclical nature of the problem was due to the executive committees (responsible for the smooth running of the union) changing, compounded by the fact that the academic year for most nursing students is different from that of other students. Eventually the message to recognise the differences that make the pre-registration nursing course so unique was received and significant progress has now been made in a fairly short period of time. It is important that differences are recognised so that the individual problems can be addressed and existing services adapted to meet needs.

Equally important is the input of nursing students to the students' union structures. This student group is renowned for not having direct involvement with the running of their students' unions, leaving them vulnerable to assumption and misunderstanding. Without a voice present in the students' union, nursing students tend to remain under-represented, despite usually being the largest single student group within the system.

STUDENTS' UNION WELFARE

The welfare officer of the local SU has the remit of providing welfare services to all students, and this includes student nurses. However, nursing students need to be aware that the complexities of the pre-registration education system have disadvantaged nursing students and the SU when dealing with welfare issues. The extended academic year and clinical placements make it difficult for nursing students to access welfare fully and for welfare officers to plan services that suit. Again, the input of nursing students is essential to making progress in this area.

To access university welfare systems, personal tutors will be able to guide individual students and information should be in the course handbook given to all new students. Prospective students can find out about welfare systems from course literature or from staff at the faculty. There may even be a member of faculty staff with the remit of facilitating this.

Hospital or clinical environment based welfare is not normally accessible for nursing students, with confusion surrounding who is responsible for the students' welfare. Any student needing help should have access to details of the 'link tutor', who will be a lecturer with responsibilities for maintaining links with the clinical placement concerned. Shift patterns can pose problems here, but systems should be in place to ensure that university staff can be contacted at any time. This is very important should a student feel that their mentor is not the most suitable person to help, or has not been able to help.

Mentors should have all the details necessary to assist students with this and there should be no reasons for lengthy delays in contacting university staff. And if all of these systems are absent or ineffective, then why not suggest some alternatives or improvements? Your faculty management will listen to any well thought out suggestions that can improve systems designed to support students.

COUNSELLING

There are several sources of counselling available for students. Access to university based counselling can be via specific named lecturers or the students' union. However, actually getting this may take some time due to waiting lists, often in excess of six weeks. Obviously, this is unacceptable for students in need of help that may arise from a crisis situation and systems should be in place that can assist students. Many students' unions run crisis or help telephone lines that can provide basic counselling services. Times and levels of such services will be available in the students' union handbook.

For nursing students, however, there is the added problem of such services not being available during out of term times (based on the university degree programmes). Your own department will have details of the available services during and out of university term times. Your students' union will have details of other services available for students in need of counselling, be it formal or informal. If there is a faculty-based member of staff with a welfare remit, he or she too will be able to provide information.

Student members of the Royal College of Nursing can access counselling services by telephone or face to face. Details of this member service can be obtained through RCN Direct on 0345 726 100 (24 hours).

HEALTH PROMOTION

Health promotion is an integral part of the nursing profession. As such, you would expect nursing students to be among the healthiest of all! Practising what must be preached is not always very easy, and nursing students, along with their qualified colleagues, have a long way to go in ideal health. Smoking among nurses is higher that the national average, and students don't escape this. For students, there must be input in terms of health promotion.

It has to be reiterated that the difficulties faced in delivering services to nursing students leave the group vulnerable. Missing out on opportunities to understand the risks of smoking, unsafe sex and meningitis, for example, is not acceptable. And no, there is no automatic filtering in of this information just because these students are being educated as health professionals. If anything, the assumption that nursing students will know better than any other student group is a dangerous one that indicates the need for services to be in place from an early point in the course.

Immunisations that are required (most notably Hepatitis B) should be provided prior to a student's first clinical placement. This is a critical factor that should be addressed as part of an overall health promotion package that should be tailored to the needs of nursing students. Often students are charged for these immunisations. Student activist groups, students' unions or professional organisations, such as the RCN, do not consider this normal or acceptable. Where this is happening, students should take positive action to stop such practices that only add to student hardship.

Uniforms are linked with health and safety for nursing students, as with all qualified staff, and there is much literature and debate surrounding this. A badly designed or fitting uniform can hamper moving and handling techniques.

Uniforms are a hot issue with nursing students, with certain universities charging for the provision of them. At the time of writing, the Association of Nursing Students had made significant progress in ensuring that this practice does not continue. The government stance on this issue is that universities are granted contracts and payments for the provision of pre-registration nursing education and that the contract includes the provision of uniforms. As such, any nursing student that is charged for uniforms should contact his or her students' union or professional representative who will be able to report this to the relevant people.

Alternatively, individual students can write to their member of parliament, or attend one of the advertised MP surgeries and inform government that way. This is also a useful way to bring the attention of government to some of the many issues faced by nursing students.

MONEY

This is always an issue for any student, yet for nursing students, particularly those on the diploma course, the payment of a non means-tested bursary has caused a lot of problems that are now well recognised. Many problems surround the eligibility of a student when attempting to claim state benefits or hardship funds. For the single student with a bursary, most additional sources of money are not accessible, and for those with dependants, the bursary affects the levels of benefits or funds dramatically.

Nursing students on four-year degree programmes now receive a means-tested bursary that replaced the local authority grant system. Although this bursary payment allows students access to the student loans system, the loans are at a lower maximum level than for any other course of study leading to a degree.

It is the experience of nursing students that the bursary, as it exists, is simply not enough to meet the needs of those that depend on it. The bursary is meant to provide for day-to-day living expenses, including accommodation and travel, but students remain in the difficult situation of having to take on additional part time work to supplement their income. This is often at the expense of valuable study time – time that is even scarcer during clinical placements!

FINDING OUT MORE

Contact your students' union for details of any nursing activists/representatives at your university, or look out for their details on college notice boards. The students' union can also help you to establish new groups that you think may be needed.

Student members of the Royal College of Nursing can contact local representatives, officers and student stewards via RCN Direct (0345 726 100). There are many ways to become involved with ANS activities and gain the most from your student membership.

USEFUL WEBSITE ADDRESSES

United Kingdom Central Council for Nursing, Midwifery and Health Visiting
www.ukcc.org.uk

Welsh National Board for Nursing, Midwifery and Health Visiting
www.wnb.org.uk

English National Board for Nursing, Midwifery and Health Visiting
www.enb.org.uk

National Board for Nursing, Midwifery and Health Visiting for Scotland
www.nbs.org.uk

National Board for Nursing, Midwifery and Health Visiting for Northern Ireland
www.n-i.nhs.uk/NBNI/index.htm

The Royal College of Nursing of the United Kingdom
www.rcn.org.uk

National Union of Students
www.nus.org.uk

National Union of Students, Northern Ireland
www.nus-usi.org.uk

National Union of Students, Wales
www.enablis.co.uk/nus.wales

Nursing Portal (search engine)
www.nursing-portal.com

9 The Net – information technology in healthcare

Ken Campbell

Amid the discussions on the effects of Project 2000 on nurse training very little attention has been paid to an area likely to have wide-reaching and long-lasting impact. Nurses emerging from full time student status are likely to be more confident in their use of computers as tools than any previous generation. This is perhaps fortunate in light of the anticipated introduction of the electronic patient record (EPR) and the National Electronic Library of Health (NeLH), both of which are likely to impact greatly on day-to-day clinical and nursing practice.

This outline of information technology is intended to give an overview of the types of software available, the uses for which each type is best suited and the use of the Internet and the World Wide Web as resources for student and practising nurses. There is no coverage of hardware (computers and their accessories) for two reasons. First is that all too often the whole topic of information technology becomes heavily biased towards the technology and one forgets that the central concern should be the information and what can usefully be done with it. A new concept is emerging of knowledge management – that of active management of information rather than passive consumption. Second is that in most cases the hardware to be used is likely to be determined by your college or employer. As an end-user you are more likely to have at least some influence over the software you will be using than the hardware.

Types of software

Word processor

At its simplest level the word processor is a text-handling program used for preparing and editing documents. If your requirements are no more complex than this then the programs NotePad and WordPad (included as part of the Windows operating system) may meet all your needs. If you want a little more sophistication there are several very good freeware text editors which can be downloaded from the Web or found on the CD-ROMs given away on the front of many computing magazines. All of these are restricted to preparation of simple text documents.

The more typical word processor is a very capable text editor but offers a number of additional features. Virtually all modern word processors will offer the ability to create tables (which can include simple mathematical formulae). Most modern word processing software also offers mail merge – a tool that can create 'personalised' letters from a standard form letter and a file of names and addresses. It is mail merge that is responsible for those irritating junk letters that tell you that you may have won a fabulous prize. With a little imagination the mail merge facility can function as a simple database and produce reports based on the content of a data file.

Spreadsheet

Spreadsheets were the original business application that brought computers onto the desk and away from the central data processing concept. A spreadsheet is essentially the electronic equivalent of a huge sheet of squared paper. Each square can hold a number or a formula and the power of the spreadsheet lies in the ability of the formulae to manipulate the contents of the squares (cells). Spreadsheets can be used for very sophisticated numerical analysis and forecasting; from the smallest business to major multinational corporations the spreadsheet is an invaluable tool. Most modern spreadsheets have an extensive range of built-in statistical functions and can be used for a variety of clinical studies. For simple data sets the built-in data handling functions of a spreadsheet may be perfectly adequate. They may well be less user-friendly than dedicated database software – often it is critical exactly how the data is arranged on the spreadsheet; the program will assume the field descriptions are in a particular location.

Database management system

For more complex data sets the data handling facilities in spreadsheets or word processing programs are likely to be inadequate. There are two types of dedicated database program: flat-file and relational. A flat-file database is the electronic equivalent of an index card system. Each record in the system has its own 'card' with individual items of data contained in fields. The advantage of a flat-file database over filing cards is that the records in a database file can instantly be resorted by any field, or a subset of records can be selected based on the contents of one or more fields.

A relational database is preferred in situations where a given piece of data would be entered many times. An example would be records of named nurse care – each nurse's details will need to be entered several times and a given patient may be cared for by more than one named nurse. There is a great deal of redundancy of data and there is a risk that details may not be entered consistently on each occasion.

Nurse	Patient
Jane Bloggs, RGN	Joe Higgs
Jane Bloggs, RN	Bill Smith
June Brown	Joseph Higgs
June Brown	Pete Jenkins

Table 9.1 Example of a relational database

In the example shown Jane Bloggs appears twice but her details differ and a search for Jane Bloggs, RN would miss one entry. Similarly Joe Higgs appears twice but with differing details; a search for Joseph Higgs would miss Joe Higgs. A carelessly designed search for Jane Bloggs, RN nursing Joe Higgs would reveal no records.

In a relational database separate files would be created to hold the details for each nurse (entered only once) and each patient (again unique entries). The two files are then linked as necessary. When a new patient assignment is created the first step is to establish whether the patient and/or nurse already have entries. If either or both is not already on the system a new record is created. A relational database may be more difficult to learn to use but it will offer very sophisticated analysis techniques and for very large data sets it will create a much smaller database. More modern relational databases create links graphically by drawing lines between boxes representing the fields in each separate database and these are quite intuitive. In order to exploit fully the powerful capabilities of a modern relational database it may be necessary to learn a programming language. The database languages are usually similar to Microsoft's Visual Basic.

Presentation graphics

The impressive slides seen at scientific or clinical meetings have almost certainly been produced using one of a range of modern presentation graphics packages. These usually include a range of templates designed to facilitate creation of commonly used slide presentations, for example presenting a technical report. Presentation graphics software usually comes with a range of professionally designed templates. These templates are very widely used and your audience may well have seen them before. It is possible to create your own templates from scratch, however it is necessary to be very careful with colour combinations to ensure that text can be read easily. Probably the commonest mistake is to include too much content in a slide – the resulting small text size will be impossible to read any further back than the first two rows. If in doubt stand about six feet away from the computer monitor with the slide filling the screen – if you cannot read the content your audience will not be able to either.

It is increasingly common in modern conference centres to be able to run a slide presentation as a screen-show. This allows the use of sound, animation and video clips. If you are preparing an on-screen presentation do remember that effects which might intrigue when used sparingly will rapidly annoy your audience if used on every slide. It can quickly become very boring to have every block of text introduced one letter at a time to the sound effect of a typewriter.

Integrated suites

There are now a number of integrated suites available. These typically include a word processor, a spreadsheet program and a presentation package. Some also include a database although this is not a standard. Integrated suites, if well designed, allow the various components to be used together more easily than using separate software from different sources. When including all or part of a spreadsheet or chart or an extract from a database into a document there are two options. The data can be embedded in which case any changes made in the data will not be updated in the document. The alternative is to link the data to the original source in which case it is updated from the original source each time the document is opened. In a report it may not be desirable to have data changing each time the report is reprinted; the other potential problem with linking is that if the original source file is moved or deleted the data will be missing next time the document is opened.

SOURCES OF SOFTWARE

Commercial software

The most expensive option, commercial software, refers to the full program as marketed with manuals and usually some entitlement to technical support, although the support may be for a very limited period. Some institutions follow a policy of only allowing approved copies of full commercial software to be installed on their computers. For private users this is likely to be prohibitively expensive (programs may cost hundreds or even thousands of pounds).

Fortunately, there are perfectly legal ways to obtain the same effectiveness for a fraction of the cost. Amazingly, as a marketing ploy, software publishers often give away full copies of the last but one version of their software via the CD-ROMs mounted on the front of many computer magazines. The only omissions are the manuals, which can often be replaced with third-party books, and the technical support. A recent example contains a complete suite of software including a sophisticated word processor, a spreadsheet, a relational database and a presentation package. The suite also includes a number of accessories such as an address book and calendar. The entire software suite lacking only manuals and support was given away on the front of a PC magazine. I have commercial software valued at many thousands of pounds (at original prices) obtained in just this way and would strongly recommend keeping a keen lookout for such valuable give-aways.

At this point a warning on pirated software is in order. Not only is the purchaser of an illegal copy of a commercial program breaking the law, he or she is also running a very high risk of computer virus infections. Given the amount of grief which buying and using pirated software can cause and the ease of obtaining cheap or even free software (see below) it just is not worth it.

Shareware

Shareware is a marketing concept unique to computer software. It is as though you could walk into your local record shop, take away a copy of an album and be trusted to pay for it if you continued playing it after a trial period had ended. This approach actually works for software: no one can know how many unregistered (not paid for) versions of a given program there may be, but it is clear that enough people do register their copies to keep shareware authors in business. Many shareware programs limit functionality, by switching off certain capabilities in the unregistered version; while other programs will run perfectly for a set period, often 30 days, and then cease to work.

Shareware programs vary in price, from a few pounds to tens of pounds or occasionally more. They are invariably a great deal cheaper than their commercial equivalent. If this economic alternative is to continue it is important for users to respect the system and register their software. It is permissible, and indeed encouraged, for users to supply copies of the unregistered program to anyone they wish. To use shareware in a working environment in breach of the associated conditions or to distribute copies of the registered program is just as much against the law as using illegal copies of commercial software.

Public domain software

Some software authors write programs for the pleasure and intellectual challenge rather than as a way to make money. These authors will often release their software as public domain software. Another major source of public domain software is the US government – under Federal Law software developed with support from Federal monies must be placed in the public domain. An excellent program made available on this basis is called Epi-Info and was created as a tool for investigation of disease outbreaks. It is a very good general-purpose statistical analysis tool; among other uses it would be ideal for analysing the responses to a questionnaire.

It is important to understand that, unless explicitly otherwise stated, public domain property remains the intellectual property of the author. All that has been given up is the right to payment for use of the program.

Public domain software may legally be used and copied and supplied to others without payment of any fee. If the software author has set conditions then use is only legal so far as those conditions are complied with. If a third party attempts to commercially exploit public domain software he or she may still be liable to prosecution. An exception to this rule is a small charge for the cost of the medium (floppy disk) and for copying which is permitted.

THE INTERNET AND THE WORLD WIDE WEB

The terms Internet and Web are often used as though they are interchangeable – this is not so as the Web is just one part of the Internet. The Internet (with a capital I) is a global system which allows computers to communicate using specialised software. An internet (with a lower case i) is any set of two or more computers connected by modem or cable – an internal network for use within a company or organisation is often termed an intranet. The Internet includes facilities for electronic mail (Email), the World Wide Web and newsgroups – discussion groups, most of which are open to the public but some of which are moderated (all contributions are screened before being posted on newsgroups). Newsgroups are particularly notorious as haunts for peddlers of pornography, but it is important to realise that they also offer invaluable support groups for patients to offer mutual support. A slight modification of the newsgroup is the mailing list. This has a closed membership and is a system for mutual Email contact between groups of people with common interests. A typical example of a mailing list is the HemOnc list for anyone (patients or others) with an interest in haematological oncology.

The Internet was originally created by the US military as a means of keeping open communications after a limited nuclear exchange. The system is now available to anyone who has a computer, a modem (a device which allows computers to communicate via the telephone system) and an account with an Internet Service Provider (ISP). An ISP is a company that provides the software and the connections needed to identify your computer to other computers on the Internet and which allows you to connect to other computers. There are now many ISPs offering free connection to the Internet (financed by taking a small cut of the phone charge and sometimes by advertisements). By registering with one of these free ISPs it is possible to connect to the Internet for no more than the cost of a local rate phone call.

The World Wide Web is a system, operating as part of the Internet, which allows authors to create pages with text and images, sounds and video. These Web pages are viewed using software called a browser. Several different types of Web browser are now available free of charge – new computers virtually all include a Web browser as part of the standard set-up. Older browsers may have limited abilities to view complex Web pages, but courteous Web page designers attempt to make sure that their pages are readable even on very old browsers used on slow machines. This is particularly important when using the Web as a means to distribute patient information, an increasingly common practice.

There are many different resources contained within the Internet and it is becoming common practice for articles and academic papers to reference material from such sources. There are now several academic journals that exist on the Web but have no printed counterpart.

Email	Equivalent to personal communication.
Newsgroups	Non-permanent, equivalent to non peer-reviewed journals, archived on the Web.
Web pages	Need to assess reliability and stability of source. If there is a print version always give this as the reference.

Table 9.2 Character of Internet and Web resources

CITING ELECTRONIC RESOURCES IN ACADEMIC WRITING

There are several different conventions for citing electronic resources, that is papers from the Internet or the Web. It is likely that eventually all standard formats for citing academic references (Harvard, Vancouver and so on) will include directions for electronic resources – the Harvard system has already included instructions, but at present it is necessary when writing for college or university or for publication to establish the appropriate format. The Web is so vast in extent that it is far beyond the scope of this chapter to summarise the available resources. A monograph entitled 'The Internet: a Perennial Resource for Nurses' (Heenan, 1999) offers a useful overview for nurses and nursing students. A few other potentially useful sites are listed below. Although the Web is inherently

Student survival guide

changeable these are all resources that are liable to remain available for the foreseeable future.

An Internet Guide for the Health Professional, 2nd Edition, 1996
http://newwindpub.com/medguide/table.htm

World Wide Web Virtual Library of Nursing
http://milkman.cac.psu.edu/~dxm12/wwwlibng.html

NURSE
http://www.csv.warwick.au.uk:8000/default.html

American Journal of Nursing company
http://www.ajn.org

National Institute of Nursing Research
http://www.nih.gov/ninr

Nursing and child-related resources
http://pegasus.cc.ucf.edu/~wink/home.html

Medline
http://www.nlm.nih.gov

Biomednet
http://www.biomednet.com/db/medline

Nursing Portal (search engine)
http://www.nursing-portal.com

British Nursing News Online
http://nurse-nurses-nursing.com

FINA
http://fina-nursing.com

References

Heenan, A. (1999) *The Internet: a Perennial Resource for Nurses*. London: NT Books.

10 The Pure Hell of St Trinian's – academic hints and tips

Janet Hesketh

The aim of this chapter is to provide advice on coping with the academic side of your nurse training.

In order to care effectively for patients, nurses need to understand the rationale that underpins their clinical practice. Caring without understanding and knowledge can be counterproductive and dangerous. The elderly lady recovering from a hip operation will not regain her independence if you do everything for her, and the young man may die if you don't recognise the significance of his slowing pulse rate. A nurse must be able to distinguish the significant from the ordinary and routine, and must use his or her knowledge of human biological, psychological and social functioning to assess the complex health needs of children, adults, families and communities. You cannot hope to provide effective care for your patients without the underpinning theoretical knowledge.

Unlike most other professions, nursing has drawn on knowledge from other disciplines, such as physiology, medicine, pharmacology and microbiology, as well as specific nursing knowledge, to provide its theoretical underpinnings. This means that as student nurses you are expected to cover a much broader curriculum than students following single discipline courses, such as psychology or biology.

Over the last 20 years there has been a tremendous growth in our knowledge and understanding of human development, human behaviour and the disease processes that threaten human life and well being. You only have to compare the size of textbooks from the 1960s to those of today to see what I mean. It is no longer possible for you to learn everything you will need to know about nursing during your initial training. The aim of pre-registration courses is to introduce you to the main concepts and ideas and give you the study skills to build on this knowledge throughout the rest of your career.

However, if this knowledge is to be useful to you in practice it has to be applied to the clinical situation. Theory and practice are two sides of the same coin – they should not be separated. Try thinking of your patients and the clinical areas you visit as animated textbooks. When you are looking after a patient with chronic obstructive airways disease try to imagine what is happening in his or her lungs and blood stream to produce the symptoms you are observing from the outside. In lectures, when you are learning about the cardiovascular system and heart disease try to relate the information you are being taught to real patients with real symptoms that you have nursed on the wards and in the community.

Learning is about taking 'on board' new ideas and new information, integrating the new material with your existing knowledge to create new understandings, which you can then utilise to help you interpret new situations and experiences.

Study skills will help you to manage information and make the most of every learning opportunity.

The theoretical component of your course is designed to help you understand your patients/clients from a biopsychosocial perspective by introducing you to a range of ideas and concepts through the use of lectures, discussions and seminars and through your own reading of appropriate books and journals.

LECTURES

A lecture is a formal presentation on a particular topic and is traditionally the most widely used teaching method in higher education. It is most commonly used with large groups of students. The lecturer presents material, accompanied by overhead transparencies (OHTs), slides, videos or demonstrations while the students make notes.

Unfortunately, unless the lecturer and/or the material is particularly interesting, most students find it difficult to concentrate for more than about 20 minutes before their minds start to wander and they lose interest. Most lecturers are aware of this and try to break the lecture up by using questions or activities to try to keep their audience involved and attentive. However, there are things that you as a student can do to make sure you get the most out of the lecture.

Lectures are given to help 'frame' your understanding of a particular topic, to present an argument, a point of view, to stimulate your interest, or to show how different ideas and concepts can be integrated into clinical practice. They do this by 'talking' you through the material, using their tone of voice, expression and body language to give emphasis, meaning and impact to ideas and concepts. Some lecturers are better at doing this than others. Also, some topics lend themselves better to this approach than others. But whatever the lecturer's style or the subject you will get more out of the lecture if you can get actively involved in it.

Start by reviewing your existing knowledge on the topic or try familiarising yourself with the subject by reading the appropriate chapter in a textbook or reading a journal article on the subject. Don't worry if you don't understand it all; that's where the lecture can help clarify your thinking. But try to make sure you have some idea of the terms and concepts that are likely to be included.

Most courses include lists of learning outcomes which specify what you are expected to have learnt by the end of the course or module. Identify the learning outcomes for the session and focus on them. Ask yourself how the material from the lecture will help you be a better nurse or achieve a good grade in your next assignment. We all learn better when we see the relevance of the material for ourselves.

Finally, be an active listener. Don't just sit back and accept what the lecturer is saying – be critical, ask yourself questions. Does this fit in with what I already know? Can I relate what is being said to my experiences? Believe it or not you have time to do this. Most people speak at about 125 to 175 morphemes (the smallest component of speech) per minute, but we can think at 400 to 800 morphemes per minute. So you have spare thinking capacity while you are listening. Unless you use this time to evaluate what the speaker is saying and make links to your existing knowledge, this spare thought time gets used for unrelated activities, such as day dreaming or doodling.

Student survival guide

DISCUSSIONS, TUTORIALS AND SEMINARS

These are similar to lectures, but are usually less formal and involve smaller numbers of students. Again the purpose is to enhance your understanding of a particular topic, but it will only work if you play an active part in the process. Don't accept everything the lecturer says – challenge, question, get involved. Your opinions and experiences have as much validity as everyone else's in the group and it is only through sharing experiences and exchanging ideas that we all learn – including the lecturers!

Being able to make fast, accurate, legible notes is a skill that will be useful to you throughout your nursing career and not just while you are studying. Being able to produce an accurate summary of a meeting or a discussion, being able to write a concise report or summarise a patient's history are skills that develop from effective note taking.

There are three basic ways of noting information:

- sequentially – in the order in which the information is given (see Fig 10.1);
- patterned – according to a structure which the lecturer imposes (see Fig 10.2);
- mapped – according to a conceptual structure that makes sense to you (see Fig 10.3).

Sequential notes

Factors influencing development

Genes – inheritance – nature

Environment – nurture

Inherited factors
- Physical features
- Personality and behaviour
- Multifactoral inheritance
- Environmental factors
- Class
- Gender
- Culture and ethnicity
- Location

Fig 10.1

The Pure Hell of St Trinian's – academic hints and tips

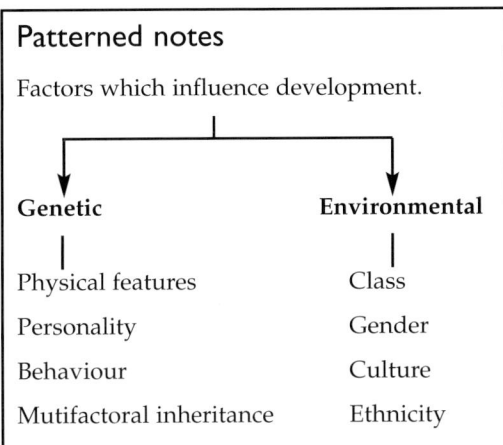

Fig 10.2

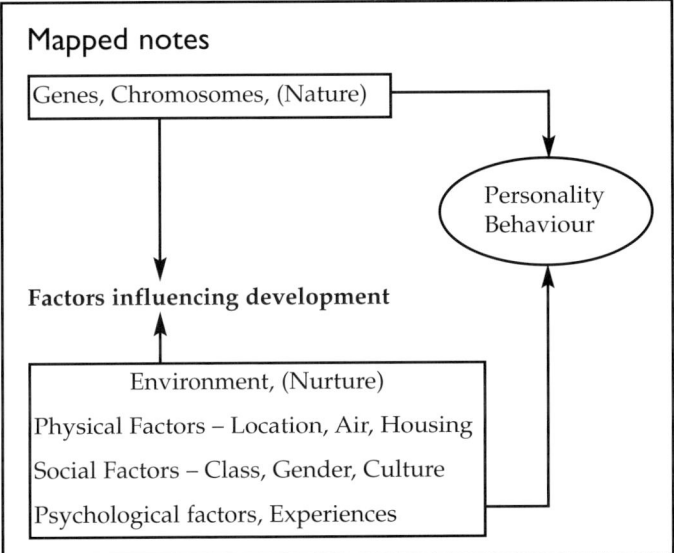

Fig 10.3

Alternatively you may have developed your own method. The exact method you choose to make notes is unimportant – what is important is that it is effective and works for you.

Making notes from books and journals

The purpose and process is exactly the same as making notes from a lecture, the difference being you can do it at your own pace. When making notes from books or journals always start by noting down the complete reference of the source. From personal experience I can assure you that there is nothing more frustrating than trying to trace the source of a particular piece of information from the library when you can't remember from where you got it.

When using books don't feel you have to read them from cover to cover – be selective, use the index to find the relevant information. You can skim read by reading the first couple of sentences in each paragraph to identify the appropriate section of the text. If you don't feel you understand exactly what the author is saying, try reading about the same topic in a different book.

When making notes from your own textbooks or using photocopies of text you can highlight sections of text as you read or make comments in the margins. However, it can be difficult re-reading text that has been highlighted. Alternatively you can mark the text in the margins using a pencil which can be rubbed out if necessary.

Organising your notes

Once created, notes should be used. You need to design a system for filing and storing notes which allows you to access them easily.

One way to organise notes is by subject area. Create a file for each subject containing lecture notes, journal articles, newspaper cuttings, reference and book lists – in fact, any information relating to that subject. Alternatively you can file by type of information, so you would have a file for lecture notes, a file for journal articles and so on. Again the actual method is unimportant as long as it works for you and you can find the information when you need it.

One method I would not recommend was that adopted by my eldest son. He filed the research notes for his dissertation all over his bedroom floor. It worked well until I wanted to tidy up!

Once you have organised your material, you can then use it to help you in preparing essays and assignments or in revising for examinations.

Writing essays and assignments

The purpose of asking students to write essays and assignments is to enable assessment of their progress in and understanding of a particular topic. The process of writing also helps you to deepen and consolidate your knowledge and understanding of the material.

Academic writing is a skill which you can learn and in which you can improve your performance through practice.

The stages of essay writing

1. Taking in the title.
2. Gathering material.
3. Generating ideas.
4. Planning.
5. Writing the first draft.
6. Reviewing.
7. Final draft.
8. Submission.

It is important that you make sure you answer the question or address the issues in the title because, however well written or well referenced your work is, it will not pass if it does not fulfil the assessment criteria.

Start by identifying the key words or issues in the title, and make sure you understand exactly what the examiners require.

Key words used in titles

Compare	– Look for similarities between components or categories within the topic area.
Contrast	– Look for differences.
Criticise	– Make judgements on an issue, and support the judgements with evidence from literature.
Define	– Illustrate the meaning of a topic.

Describe	–	Create a verbal picture of a topic.
Differentiate/ Distinguish	–	Highlight the differences between subjects.
Discuss	–	Explore by a process of argument. Argue for or against. Weigh up the possible implications of an issue.
Evaluate	–	Appraise the issue in question, with reference to its purpose or intention or effectiveness.
Explain	–	Clarify component parts of an issue or topic.
Illustrate	–	Give a graphic account of the issue or process.
Justify	–	Defend or support an argument or viewpoint.
Outline	–	Produce a framework that encompasses the issue/topic.
Summarise	–	Bring together the main points of an issue, and express the implications in relation to the topic area.

Gathering material

You should always start your preparation by reading around your topic area looking for ideas. Use books, journals, the Internet, databases, newspapers, magazines, TV programmes – anything that will help you generate ideas. Databases like Medline and Cinahl can yield vast amounts of information which you may not be able to access, so it may be useful to start by restricting your search to material you have available locally.

Alternatively you can use the 'hard copies' of the index to look under specific headings for information. Journals are excellent sources of information, but it is important to recognise that different journals are written for different audiences and this is reflected in the type of articles they publish. For example *Nursing Times* and *Nursing Standard* are aimed at a general nursing audience and contain news, features and articles of general interest. The *Journal of Advanced Nursing* and the *British Journal of Clinical Nursing* contain papers of academic interest or research reports. There are several journals that focus on specific areas of nursing practice and contain news, articles and research relevant to their specialist area. Journals which are published monthly normally include an index of authors and subjects in the last issue of each year and these can be a very useful as a quick source of relevant articles to get you started.

The more academic journals, like the *Journal of Advanced Nursing*, regularly publish reviews of published literature on a specific topic. These are normally excellent guides to the topic area and well worth photocopying. When you have found articles relevant to your assignment, always check the reference list to see where they got their information from as there is a good chance it will be relevant to your assignment as well. You will need to look at 'classic' work as well as recent work in order to get a balanced view of the topic.

Generating ideas

Once you have read round the topic you are then in a position to generate your own ideas and thoughts on the subject. Although you will be using other people's ideas and research, it is the way you link and use these ideas that makes it your work. If you copy chunks of text from someone else's work you may well be accused of plagiarism. You must always acknowledge your sources both in the text of your assignment and in the reference list.

Planning

This is where you make a rough list of the points you want to make and then try to arrange them into a logical order. As a tutor, this is the point at which I like to meet with my students to discuss their ideas. It is much easier to make changes at this stage than later in the process.

Writing the first draft

In writing the first draft it is more important to get the ideas and content down on paper than to get the words exactly right. If you get stuck with something just indicate what you want to say and move on to the next paragraph. Whenever possible, use a word processor because of the ease with which it allows you to edit and move text. If you are handwriting your work, I would advise only writing on one side of the paper and using a new sheet for each section. Again this allows you space for editing.

Most essays or assignments are divided into three sections: introduction, main body and conclusion.

Student survival guide

Introduction

This section should indicate what you think the question means, and how you intend to answer it. You should give the rationale for including particular material in your answer and show how it relates to the question. The introduction usually comprises no more than 10% of the total essay.

Main body

This is where you develop your argument, present your evidence and analyse and discuss information. Each point you make should be supported by appropriate evidence in the form of at least one reference or quotation. The number of references you use should relate to the number of points in your argument. Your essay should not be a list of quotations from other authors loosely joined together. Be critical – don't accept everything you read just because it was published in a book or journal. Analyse what you read, challenge it, and if you can find evidence from your clinical experience or another author to back you up, don't be frightened to use it.

In academic writing there are no marks for literary style or use of metaphor. Make your essay as readable as possible. Try to avoid long convoluted sentences. Each paragraph should be complete in itself. The first sentence in a paragraph should set the scene: it can be a major point, with the rest of the paragraph used to explore, expand or justify it or you can use the first sentence to pose a question and answer it in the rest of the paragraph. It is important to remember that the reader cannot see into your mind so you need to 'signpost' your argument throughout the essay by making obvious the connections between points and referring back to the title to show how a particular point fits into your overall argument.

Conclusion

The conclusion should draw the threads of your argument together and emphasise the main points. It should be based on the evidence you have provided in the main body of the assignment. Don't introduce new material in the conclusion but do show how the discussion has answered the question set in the title.

When students ask me to look at their first drafts I prefer to see the whole assignment, regardless of how 'rough' it is, rather than just pieces. I see my role as being to point out the weaknesses in the argument and offer advice on strengthening the discussion rather than simply correcting spelling and grammar.

Reviewing

At this stage you need to go over the material correcting errors and omissions, finalising the wording and making sure the content is relevant. Check that you are within the required word limit.

Final draft

At this point the writing process should be over and you need to concentrate on general presentation, spelling, references and punctuation.

Submission

It is important to adhere to any guidelines you are given with regard to presentation as these are designed to assist the marking process.

PREPARING FOR EXAMINATIONS

As well as assignments most pre-registration courses include at least one written examination.

To many students, exams are the worst part of studying any course. However, they can be a useful tool for checking whether a student has acquired sufficient knowledge to be regarded as competent in that particular subject.

You should try to think of exams as a chance to demonstrate how much you have learnt, not a test of how much you don't know.

An examination sets up a framework within which you need to consolidate knowledge and skills in order to achieve a particular standard. Be honest – how much time and effort would you spend going over your notes if you didn't have an examination to prepare for?

An exam presents you with a challenge. It puts you under pressure and creates stress. During an emergency on the ward most people find they are able to concentrate solely on the task at hand. Nothing else matters. They are able to ignore everything else and focus on saving the patient's life. An exam is a way of creating a mini-crisis. It forces you to focus your attention on the course material. Exam preparation is about using that pressure and stress creatively to help you achieve your optimum performance.

Unfortunately, used negatively that stress can create its own problems and lead to poor performance in the examination.

Revising for examinations

Revision should be an active process, not simply a reading and re-reading of your notes. The object is not to memorise pages of notes but to make sure you understand the material covered in the course and can explain it in your own words. It should be planned around meaningful activities, such as answering past exam questions or creating revision notes.

Timing

How much time you allocate to your revision is up to you. It will depend on your commitments and how you like to revise. But be realistic: you can get very tired working shifts on placement and it is difficult to study effectively if you are tired. Work out how much time you have for revision and the topic areas you want to revise. Decide when you are going to study and allocate the time evenly between the topics. Remember to include time off for relaxation and reward yourself when you feel you have done well.

Creating revision notes

This is a major part of the revision process and will help you use your time more effectively. Start by looking at the notes and other information you have collected on your chosen topic areas and identify the most relevant material for your purpose. Condense and integrate this material into short notes. Extract the main points from these condensed notes into a single summary sheet of headings with key points, names, references and so on for that topic.

Depending on the type of exam it may be possible to take the main headings from the topic summary sheets to produce a single summary sheet which outlines the main points of the subject. This works best with single subjects, for example sociology or psychology, but it might be useful to try to produce single summary sheets for broad topics, for example surgical nursing or human development. Condensing material into manageable chunks like this makes it easier to memorise and the knowledge can be used in the actual exam to help plan your answers.

Answering past exam questions

This is a very useful revision activity. Most schools keep copies of old exam papers for students to use for revision. You don't need to write out the answer in full every time, just concentrate on the planning stage and produce an outline answer. Then either ask a tutor to have a look at it or refer back to the course material to see if you have left anything out. Don't try learning model answers by rote; you will need to adapt your answer to the specific question in the exam and you will be penalised if you don't do this.

On the day of the exam

Try to approach the exam day calmly, take your time over getting ready and leave yourself plenty of time to get to the exam. If you do have a crisis on the day, don't panic, there are solutions to most problems and there are usually contingency plans for dealing with the more common problems, such as traffic delays and sickness.

Answering the question

Always start by reading the paper and tick the questions you know something about it. If the sight of a blank sheet of paper makes you 'freeze' start writing even if it is only to write the question out. Tackle your best question first but make your sure you have read the question and know exactly what it is asking. Underlining the key words can help. Take time to plan your answer before you start writing. A well-planned answer will ensure you get the main points down in a logical order. Everything you write should be relevant to the question. There are no marks for irrelevant material.

Plan how much time you have for each answer and don't overrun. The first 50% of the marks allocated for a particular question are usually fairly easy to get if you know the basic material. The second 50% and especially the last 25% are the hardest to get; it has to be a really exceptional answer to be awarded marks in the highest range. It is always better to go for three reasonable answers than try to compensate two poor answers with one good one.

And finally, try to write legibly. When an examiner is reading a lot of scripts it makes the marking process much harder if he or she is struggling to read what has been written on the exam paper.

Exams are designed to be passed by the majority of the students taking them – if they don't there is something wrong with the exam not the students.

PRESENTATIONS

After exams the next most traumatic experience for students seems to be making presentations.

A useful strategy for helping students learn is to ask small groups of students to go off and research a particular topic and then present their findings to the rest of the group. Most students seem to enjoy the first bit but seem to dread standing up in front of the group to present their findings.

If you are asked to make a presentation, start by making notes exactly as you would for an essay or an assignment. Put the main points into a logical order and use this as a framework for your presentation. You can put the main points on a poster or an OHT to act as a guide for what you want to say.

When it comes to speaking, remember that the rest of the students are on your side – they don't want to do it either, so take a deep breath and get on with it. Try talking to your audience rather than reading from your notes, as you will get a better response. Keep what you want to say simple and direct and don't put too much information on your OHT or poster.

The skills you learn during your training should be the foundation for your learning throughout the rest of your career.

I hope this chapter has been of some help to you and I wish you good luck with your studies.

Acknowledgements

In writing this chapter I have drawn on my own experience, both as a student and a tutor, and a variety of learning materials from various sources, including the Open University, Andrew Northedge's excellent 'The Good Study Guide' and the study skills package we use in the Faculty of Health Studies, University of North Wales, Bangor.

Recommended reading

There are several good books on study skills that include exercises and activities to help you practise different skills. Books are very personal, so I would suggest you find one that appeals to you and try that.

Buzan, T. (1982) *Use your head*. London: BBC.

Freeman, R. (1991) *Mastering Study Skills*. 2nd Edition. Basingstoke: Macmillan.

Maslin-Prothero, S.E. (1997) *Bailière's Study Skills for Nurses*. London: Bailière-Tindall.

Northedge, A. (1990) *The Good Study Guide*. Milton Keynes: Open University.

11 Up Close and Personal
– personal experiences of training

Lee Bickley, Yvonne Bossons, Jessica Cudmore and Paul Smith Roberts

This enigmatic title opens the door into a world where commitment towards a given vocation far outweighs a run-of-the-mill, humdrum existence, where the changing faces of medicine and, in particular, the Health Service challenge traditional methods and open new frontiers in the world of nursing. Here are four nurses' stories…

My name is Yvonne Bossons and I am a 26-year-old staff nurse employed at the Countess of Chester Hospital. For the past three years I have worked in the theatre recovery unit at the hospital, where two days are never the same and where we are witness to a varied and wide-ranging schedule of operations and subsequent recovery procedures.

My education consisted of attendance at a village primary school. I moved onto the local comprehensive where I passed nine GCSEs and then onto sixth form college where I studied A Levels.

After leaving sixth form college I applied for nurse training. However, I discovered that the next intake would be a minimum of an 18-month wait, so I embarked on a series of work experience ventures that ranged from working in retail to work experience at the local hospital.

My application for nurse training was successful and I commenced in September 1992 at both the Countess of Chester and Arrow Park hospitals.

Up Close and Personal – personal experiences of training

The members of my training group were the pioneers of a new concept in nursing training within the Cheshire/Mersey region. Titled Project 2000, 82 students set out on what was to become an exciting, yet difficult journey.

In the initial stages of the course there were many teething problems, although these in the main can be attributed to the lack of history that all new courses face. The majority of problems stemmed from unclear curriculum timetables and individual concerns over agreed objectives that led to unease about what was actually required. I personally felt a resistance from the existing hospital staff, as I was an academic student and not an internal applicant who had started out on the first rung of the ladder.

One of the worst experiences during my training period occurred when I was on an elderly medical ward. On this occasion I was told not to answer the telephone, as I had 'no practical experience.' On reflection I now view this with a degree of wry humour. However, out of the many placement areas I visited, the majority of them were extremely relevant and allowed me to marry the knowledge I had learned in the classroom to the hands-on, practical experience. It was this that allowed me to fulfil my stated objectives.

The pressure of being in the first intake of Project 2000 in my locality took its toll early, with a significant percentage of student dropouts. The major conclusive factors of this can be attributed to both individual study time and the financial pressures facing many students, having to live on a limited budget.

However, for myself the sheer determination to achieve my set goals and to fulfil my career ambitions enabled me to complete a successful three-year training period and to achieve a diploma in my chosen career.

Having completed the course my next hurdle was to find suitable vacancies within a hospital environment. I found vacancies in various departments, but I felt my niche was in surgical areas and I was fortunate to find a position in theatre recovery. I was subsequently asked to attend an interview, recruited and I began my new role immediately. After four years post-registration, I am now a Theatre Recovery Sister within another trust.

Taking the time to reflect on my career, I believe the initial problems we faced at the onset of the course are now far outweighed by both my knowledge of medical issues and the experiences of life that I have gained from three years of detailed study and placement.

In today's society, where there is a well-publicised shortfall of nurses joining the Health Service, I would strongly recommend people to choose what is a vocation and not just another career option. Having seen this new project from its initial conception through to its completion, I would stand testimony to the fact that the sacrifices that have to be made do produce a positive and very satisfying outcome.

Yvonne Bossons

Prior to starting my nurse training, I had spent 19 years in the Armed Forces. Serving seven years in the Army, including two years attached to Special Forces, I served the following 12 years in the Royal Air Force. In 1995 I found myself in the position of being a single parent, looking after my eight-year-old daughter.

I was discharged from the RAF in March 1996. However, I did not have any definite plans for work at that time. I eventually decided that I wanted to become a psychiatric nurse. Applying to the local school of nursing and midwifery I was accepted as a mature student and started my training in September 1996 at the age of 40.

The first few months of my training were fraught with problems, the main one being financial hardship. Unused to a *very* low salary, I was 'forced' into working in the private sector of nursing during my study days, off duty and evenings off work/college. Childcare was also a major problem. The majority of money I earned was spent on child minding care. Fortunately my ailing elderly mother lives close by, and she tried to help out whenever she was physically able to.

Domestic problems aside, I found the first months of the common foundation programme (CFP) took some getting used to – not so much the academic side of things, more the practical clinical placements. I understood when I started the Project 2000 course that I would be expected to 'learn from scratch' the skills that the eventual trained nurse must learn, prior to registration. However, I found the attitude of some of the trained nursing staff on the wards to be quite patronising. So much so that at times I found myself being treated as a complete imbecile.

Up Close and Personal – personal experiences of training

However, I quickly learned to expect that kind of treatment and accepted it as part of the training. Having the middle management skills and qualifications gained in the forces, I speedily overcame those petty obstacles and focused my attention on the tasks ahead.

After working full time on clinical placements, I had to go home, prepare dinner for myself and my daughter, load the washing machine, wash up, do the ironing, vacuum clean, tidy the house and so on. By about 9.30pm I had the academic homework still to look forward to. That is to say, revision, writing essays and completing directed study homework. By around 1.30am I was usually ready for bed.

I have qualified... just!

Paul Smith Roberts

I decided that I wanted to be a nurse following a summer working in a nursing home on the edge of Dartmoor. It was a wonderful place where I really enjoyed working. I thought that people trained to be a nurse in hospital, and I had plans to go to university, so I carried on with my plans and hoped to train to be a nurse when I finished my chemistry degree. Chemistry, however, did not meet my expectations, so I scanned the prospectus for an alternative course and discovered that I could study nursing. I went to see my personal tutor to discuss transferring courses to do the nursing degree. He refused to help me stating that no student of his would leave to study nursing. He said that he would be pleased for me to transfer to study medicine, but not nursing. I definitely did not want to study medicine, so I went about transferring courses by myself: I have never looked back!

I had wanted to go to university for as long as I can remember – it was the lifestyle that I wanted as well as the education. It was my first time leaving home and I imagined that I would be terribly homesick. Instead I found great friends and had a fantastic time. The social life in university halls in the first year is second to none – we lived it up all year (and then worked all summer to pay off overdrafts!).

The nursing degree at Southampton was excellent. There were 20 girls in our group, so it was a small cohort, and we all got on really well. In the first year we had very little clinical content – a maximum of one day a

Student survival guide

week. As a consequence we did not feel like nurses at all until later in the course when we spent some more time on the wards. We had supernumerary status for the whole four years; this was the best way to learn for both us students and the patients. We could take on what we felt able to and be supervised and taught at the same time. It seemed to work very well.

The course was hard going. We had to complete four 3000-word essays every 10 weeks and we had a biohealth exam at the end of each 10-week term. This clashed with our non-nursing friends who led us astray most nights by encouraging us to party instead of study. The timetable was also more gruelling with nine to five lectures most days, unlike most of our friends, one of which had only eight hours of lectures per week!

I became involved with the Royal College of Nursing Association of Nursing Students (ANS) in my third year. I was elected as vice chair of the ANS and continued to work for them for three years. It was a great way to meet students from other colleges and share experiences. We also felt that we made a great difference to students' lives through various campaigns, such as increasing the bursary and improving nursing accommodation. The RCN conferences are excellent for meeting people, getting inspired and getting hung over. I learnt so much from the RCN and would recommend everyone to get actively involved.

The best part of the training was finally becoming a nurse. It is a job that I love doing as I feel that I can really make a difference to people's experience of hospital. It is hard work, poorly paid, yet very rewarding and at the moment I would not do anything else.

Since qualifying in 1992 I worked on a trauma ward for six months and A&E for a year before heading to London to complete my paediatric training at Great Ormond Street. Being a post-registration student was an experience that I did not enjoy, for many reasons, although now I am very pleased to be caring for children and their families. I have always taken my commitment to nursing seriously both at work and outside of work. I got elected on to the UKCC Council in April 1998 for a five year post and have been learning a great deal about the politics of nursing. I also work for *Nursing Times* as a consultant editor. I firmly believe the more that you put into life the more you get out of it!

Jessica Cudmore

Up Close and Personal – personal experiences of training

07.15 on a bleak and windswept Sunday morning I found myself on the bus from the halls of residence to the hospital. I didn't even know there was a seven o' clock in the morning! I arrived at the hospital in plenty of time to start my first shift as a student nurse. The ward was a busy 30-bed medical ward encompassing haematology, care of the elderly and endocrinology specialities. I can remember standing in the doorway of the ward thinking 'Oh my God (or words to that effect), what have I done?'. I was first introduced to my mentor who at that moment was walking down the ward with a used bedpan. She said just to follow her for the first few hours and then when things settled down mid morning she would take me round and show me where things were. Mid morning did not happen that day as bang on 10.30 the crash bells went off and people appeared from everywhere. You would have thought half the medical staff in the hospital were there. This was my first introduction to CPR and basic life support. The rest of the day was not too bad but by 16.00 I was absolutely knackered and bewildered at how much I would have to learn in the next three years.

The course that I applied to do was a Bachelor of Nursing degree that was to be completed in three years rather than the usual four. By doing this, though, the students qualified for a bursary rather than living on the student grants and loans. On the downside, it meant that we all had a lot of work to do in a very short space of time.

The course followed that of the diploma in nursing but with the degree assignments and exams on top. At one point in the course we had an 8000-word care study to hand in and two weeks later a 3000-word research paper. This was a very trying time but, with the help of the tutors, we managed to do it.

My training took an unusual pathway in that I transferred from one college to another halfway through the course. Both colleges were within the same university but it meant starting all over again with new friends and a new hospital. This was not too bad and the friends that I made keep in touch now we have all gone our separate ways.

I now work as a theatre nurse in a specialist head and neck unit in Shropshire. I really enjoy the work and the close knit team I am a part of. I work four days a week from 08.00 to 18.30 but get three days off per week. As part of the job we have to work roughly two nights per week and one weekend in four on call. This means that we cannot be outside 30 minutes travel from the hospital and cannot have a drink at all. This can be difficult as some nights we do not get home until around midnight, but it's worth it when you see the patients going home a few days later. I hope to stay in this post for a few years and then move on to A&E or a trauma unit to get more experience of 'front line' nursing.

Lee Bickley

12 Alien Nation – the other contributors to healthcare

Jill Newman

The public perception of the NHS is one of an organisation staffed by doctors and nurses and administered bureaucratically by managers. This perception is supported by political ideology and reinforced by media rhetoric.

The medical profession can still be seen to be dominant, controlling the use of much of the NHS resources. Role expansion and job enrichment in other professions, including nursing, have caused the autonomy of the professions to increase and allowed the development of the independent practitioner who is arguably less reliant on the medical profession. The expansion of traditional roles has led to the blurring of professional boundaries. This at a time when the public and political expectations for a seamless service have led to increased multidisciplinary team working.

The existence of a wide variety of uniforms within the NHS acts not merely as a manifestation of the culture and a demonstration of the presence of 'tribalism', but also as a useful mechanism to identify the role of workers both to the patients and to fellow colleagues. In the nursing profession the uniform is frequently used to support the internal nursing hierarchy, outwardly indicating the status of the nurse to all familiar with the coding used.

Within other professions the uniform is likely to identify them for their professional background but not differentiate between grades within the profession. In these cases the name badge including job title is the usual differentiating mechanism which denotes professional status. The outward distinguishing features will assist the new nurse to identify personnel within the organisation by their role and status and reinforce the organisational culture. It will therefore be evident early in a nurse's career that many occupations have a part to play in the delivery of healthcare to the patient.

The aim of this chapter is to briefly explain the role of some of the occupations nurses are likely to encounter in the healthcare setting.

Occupational groupings

It is possible to consider many of the occupations found within the NHS as having some commonality of purpose and they can therefore be placed in sub-groups. The conventional sub-groupings used are:

- medical
- nursing and midwifery
- professional allied to medicine
- professional and technical
- administrative and clerical
- estate management
- ancillary services

Medical staff

This category includes personnel with widely differing specialisms, experience and influence brought together by the shared experience of medical training through a university school of medicine. Doctors' first experience of the NHS is usually via placements from medical schools as students.

The career pathway of doctors varies with the specialism they choose to follow but generally progression within the hospital environment is from house officer following qualification to senior house officer to specialist registrar to consultant. This route is long, with six monthly rotations at house officer and senior house officer level being common. This enables the junior doctor to gain a wide range of experience in several disciplines before specialising at the level of registrar.

The junior doctor role therefore provides both a training post for the individual and service delivery for the patient. The balance between these two functions is carefully monitored by the royal colleges to ensure quality of service can be delivered by competent and appropriately trained staff.

As has already been stated the route to consultant level is lengthy and arduous and does not appeal to all medical staff. Other non-training grades are employed within the NHS, such as staff grades and associate specialists. These are fully qualified doctors who have specialised in a particular discipline and often reached senior levels without completing the necessary qualifications to attain the post of consultant. They are usually employed for their expertise in permanent non-rotation posts within medical disciplines.

The consultant is the most senior medical grade within most hospitals. Professorial posts are found in some hospitals and these posts, together with lecturer positions, indicate medical staff with a teaching, training and/or research role in addition to their commitment to service delivery. Professorial chairs are generally awarded on the basis of clinical and academic expertise and are linked to university hospitals.

It would be wrong to give the impression that the medical profession is solely hospital based. Indeed with the shift to a primary-led health service the role of the general practitioner (GP) should not be underestimated. Junior doctors wishing to work in the primary care setting will enter a general practitioner training scheme and, on successful completion of training, proceed into GP practices or partnerships. GPs may retain links to their previous hospital training by sessional commitments either as clinical assistants or, in the case of principals in GP practice, hospital practitioners. These posts usually provide service delivery in dedicated specialities on a basis of two to three sessions per week, with the post holder expected to maintain his or her clinical skills through audit and continuous medical education.

Medical staff also have a role in health service management. At a national level the chief medical officer will advise ministers on the needs of patients, the latest medical and technological developments and so on. This advice is often based on the work of doctors specialising in public health medicine, employed by health authorities.

Within the local hospital and primary care setting the doctor's role in management is growing. The newly formed Primary Care Groups (Local Health Groups in Wales) will be chaired by a GP and will function to determine the service needs of their population. Within hospitals a directorate structure is commonplace, with each directorate led by a clinical director, usually a senior consultant from within the specialisms. The clinical director not only holds the budget and determines the strategic direction of the directorate but also advises the management on the future service needs and anticipated changes within the sphere of his or her control.

PROFESSIONS ALLIED TO MEDICINE

This grouping includes a wide variety of professions that act to provide diagnostic and therapeutic services for patients, supporting medical staff in the management of patients. The entry point for most professionals within this grouping is following a three- or four-year undergraduate training resulting in a degree in the profession and a licence to practise issued by the state registration body for the profession – the Council of Professions Supplementary to Medicine. Without state registration from the Professions Supplementary to Medicine Act, a professional cannot practise within the NHS. The career structure within these professions is hierarchical. It progresses from entry practitioner level to Senior II to Senior I; Superintendent IV/III to Superintendent II to Superintendent I; district or service head to directorate business manager.

Physiotherapists

Physiotherapists are the largest profession of this grouping and also the most widely recognised. Their role is varied and specialisation is common within departments of physiotherapy. They can be found working in health centres and GP practices as well as in highly specialised environments, such as intensive care units and spinal injury units. They are frequently involved in the management and education of patients with acute or chronic conditions, ranging from ligament injury to cystic fibrosis. Physiotherapists are increasingly working as independent professionals, prescribing and monitoring treatment regimes and discharging patients from their case loads when they deem appropriate.

Radiographers

Like physiotherapy the role of the radiographer is wide and continuing to expand. Radiographers enter the profession as graduates along two discrete routes: either diagnostic radiography or therapy radiography. Diagnostic radiographers are the greater in number and are found in all hospitals and some community hospitals. Once qualified they gain experience in a wide range of imaging techniques and may take additional postgraduate qualifications in ultrasound, computed tomography, magnetic resonance scanning, radionuclide imaging, management or radiography education.

Radiography skills are also expanding to include IV injection, barium enema examinations and casualty film reporting – all previously the remit of the radiologist. The role of the X-ray department is changing from that of simply diagnosis to include treatment and palliative care of certain patient groups. This is particularly so in the case of interventional radiology which includes vascular procedures, such as angioplasty and stent insertion, biliary and renal drainages and orthopaedic procedures to name but a few.

The work of the radiographer is closely linked to that of the medical physicist from the professional and technical staff grouping. The radiographer not only has to produce high quality diagnostic images but must also ensure that the radiation dose is minimised by establishing that the examination is justified and that appropriate techniques are adopted to achieve the lowest possible doses to the patient, staff and population as a whole.

The work of the radiographer is closely interrelated with that of medical physicists, mould room technicians and oncologists. It involves the planning and delivery of treatment in radiotherapy centres. These tend to be regionally based. A high proportion of the work does relate to cancer treatment, but not all radiotherapy is directed at malignant disease.

Occupational therapy

Occupational therapists (OTs) are highly skilled at enabling patients with mental or physical impairments to live their lives to their full potential. Their role involves assessing patients' capabilities and needs. This may be in a hospital setting but frequently takes place in a home environment so as to establish how the individual will cope at home. OTs are aware of and advise on specialised aids to assist with immobility, bathing, dressing or domestic tasks. Rehabilitation of patients following acute episodes, such as stroke or trauma, is part of the role of the occupational therapist but many of their patients receive treatment and advice on living with chronic conditions like arthritis. Therapy workshops can be found within many occupational therapy departments and are commonplace in psychiatric units. These enable aptitude for work to be assessed.

Dietitians

The role of dietitians includes the management of nutritional support for patients with many different medical conditions. They will advise patients and nursing staff with regard to diabetes, endocrine disorders, liver disease and Crohn's disease to name a very few. In assessing a patient's dietary and nutritional requirements the dietician will often work closely in a team including the clinician and nursing staff. Dietitians frequently advise catering managers of the needs for inpatient nutrition and have a health promotion function with the patients and public. Sub-specialism exists in this profession as with most of the professions allied to medicine.

Speech and language therapy

Speech and language therapists treat not only patients with speech impediments but also patients having communication difficulties due to acute or chronic conditions, such as following a stroke or in the treatment of the profoundly deaf.

This is the largest of the professions supplementary to medicine. Other professions that fall into this group include art and music therapists, orthoptists, chiropodists and optometrists. Further information on all these professions can be obtained from their appropriate professional bodies or within local hospital departments.

Members of the professions allied to medicine are frequently assisted in their work by support staff, such as helpers, who do not possess professional qualifications. They are usually in-service trained to NVQ level and provide invaluable assistance to the smooth running of services.

Professional and technical staff

This grouping includes staff generally with a scientific background and includes both scientific and technical grades. Staff in this grouping can be found in a variety of environments within the health service, ranging from rehabilitation engineering through to medical physicists and laboratory staff.

The work of the scientist can include calibration and monitoring of high tech equipment, research into the application of scientific innovations into the health service and direct patient care via patient testing in laboratories and cardiology departments.

Technicians fulfil a vital service role, often working under the guidance of a scientist. Training of technicians is important to enable them to work effectively. There is a national requirement for many to remain registered and for the services provided to be accredited. As a new nurse you are most likely to come across technicians in the cardiology department where they frequently undertake electrocardiograms, 24-hour cardiac monitoring, stress and treadmill testing, lung function tests and echocardiograms.

In the laboratory, staff are employed as medical laboratory assistants (MLAs) and medical laboratory scientific officers (MLSOs) and have the potential for career progression to chief MLSO or service head. Specialisation is common within laboratory services, the usual disciplines being biochemistry, histopathology, haematology, clinical cytology and blood transfusion services. Most large hospitals have their own pathology services but some more specialised services, such as genetic testing, may be regional.

Administrative and clerical staff

Staff in this grouping provide the supporting framework for the administrative and managerial departments needed to run the hospitals. Politicians are currently targeting this group for cuts, as it is politically desirable to demonstrate reductions in the cost of bureaucracy of the NHS. The main categories of staff in this grouping include:

- personnel staff (professional and support staff);
- finance staff, including salaries and wages personnel;

- contract and information staff;
- information technology;
- medical records;
- medical secretaries;
- clerical officers;
- receptionists;
- ward clerks;
- switchboard.

The role of these staff is to provide good communication and management of the hospital for the benefit of the patient, either directly or indirectly, and to ensure the long-term survival and reputation of the hospital.

Estate management and ancillary services

Management of the NHS estate is an enormous task in itself. Due to the historical background of capital investment in the NHS the estate is of varying ages ranging from the workhouses of the late 19th century to brand new hospitals. Not all hospitals are compactly contained within one building; many are sprawled across vast sites. In addition, clinics vary in size and location and in rural areas may be remote from central estate services.

The NHS estate also includes residential accommodation for staff, students and, increasingly, for relatives. Therefore the estate officers have a large task in managing the capital assets of the buildings and land associated with hospitals. Estate managers will usually be responsible for site maintenance, grounds maintenance, capital developments on site, employing and monitoring contractors, waste disposal, water treatment and supply, electrical supply and back-up generation, sewage, domestic services, portering and catering.

All these areas are subject to legislative and regulatory control and, since the removal of Crown Immunity in the early 1990s, the NHS has been subject to prosecution for breaches in any health and safety, building, environmental or other legislation.

The estate manager therefore needs to be extremely knowledgeable and will employ staff to assist him with the task. Some of these staff will be directly employed by the hospital but in other areas services may have been either contracted in from outside agencies or may have been contracted out as part of previous efficiency drives.

Central estate posts found in most district general hospitals will include:

- skilled tradesmen, such as plumbers, joiners and electricians;
- painters and decorators;
- boilermen;
- engineers;
- groundsmen;
- builders;
- architects and designers (brought in on a project by project basis);
- fire officer;
- health and safety officer;
- security staff.

Sub-departments of the estate function, usually termed ancillary services, include domestics, catering and portering. Domestic staff are responsible for cleaning all areas within the hospital. Competitive tendering of services during the 1980s and 1990s has led to some contracts for domestic services being placed outside the direct management of the NHS.

Closely linked with domestic services are laundry services, which may be present on site or supplied from a remote laundry. A sewing room may still be present on some sites to repair curtains and provide staff uniforms and patient clothing.

The catering manager is responsible for: ensuring efficient and high quality procurement of produce; production of nutritional inpatient meals in safe hygienic conditions; staff catering; supply of vending machines; and function catering, such as for conferences and study days. Increasingly, catering staff are under pressure to generate income.

Porters are responsible for moving patients safely around the hospital, for example between wards and theatres, outpatients to X-ray and so on. They also ensure meals are delivered to patients on wards, laundry restocked, waste disposed of, post distributed, notes circulated to required areas and drugs taken from pharmacy to ward areas. Porters take deceased patients from the wards to the mortuary. They are also used in many hospitals to direct patients, provide a security presence and respond to fire alarms. Although the portering staff are among the lowest paid in the hospital, the services they provide are essential to its smooth running on a day-to-day basis.

EXTERNAL AGENCIES

Having looked at the main occupations found within the hospital this chapter concludes with a very brief look at other bodies that are integral to the working of a hospital. These include voluntary organisations, such as the League of Friends and WRVS, local support organisations and charities, hospital radio and library services. All these organisations enlist volunteers to raise funds or work within the hospital shops or on wards, all of which contribute to improving the hospital environment for patients and staff.

In addition to this, the hospital chaplain service and parish visitors provide pastoral and religious care.

Links with social services are very important to ensure good discharge routes for many elderly patients or patients in need of support in the community. These links are frequently provided via the hospital social work service. The current move to seamless care between health and social services will mean these links will become stronger in the future.

CONCLUSION

The aim of this chapter was to give an overview of the wide variety of occupations that are necessary for the integration of healthcare provision, primarily in a hospital setting but no less importantly in the community situation. Many other occupations also contribute to the delivery of care, and failure to mention them here does not devalue their contribution. You should now be able to appreciate that the roles of all staff are essential to service delivery and without one part the others cannot function successfully.

13 Do the Right Thing –
accountability, professionalism and whistleblowing

Deborah Glover and Dr Geoffrey Hunt

ACCOUNTABILITY

That's the thing that only affects nurses when they register with the UKCC, isn't it? Well, yes and no. You are not considered to be accountable for your actions until you have qualified because, as Pennels (1997) explains: accountability is the 'requirement that each nurse is answerable and responsible for the outcome of his or her professional actions'. She goes on to say that the principle of accountability is an integral part of practice as:

- it arises from the patient's expectation that by virtue of a nurse's training and position, the nurse will be answerable to the patient while he/she is in their care;
- it arises from training and education, which explains why the notion is present in some jobs and not others. Therefore, knowledge from training is essential in order to explain why an event took place.

But you are still *responsible* for your actions. So, if the staff nurse on the ward tells you to bath a patient and you stick that patient in boiling water and scald him or her, you will be responsible for that (and in pretty hot water yourself) because, after all, that is an issue of common sense. It is not something you have to undergo training or education for.

You are also responsible for acknowledging your limitations. If you are asked to do something during the course of a clinical placement and you know nothing about it, or don't feel confident about undertaking it, you must tell the person who has delegated this to you. Trying it and hoping nothing goes wrong is not acceptable.

Here then could be the end of this chapter. Unfortunately, if I ended it here, the book would be considerably thinner than originally intended and you would feel quite conned. Therefore, the main thrust of this chapter will explain accountability in terms of how it will affect you as a qualified nurse. It is, however, worthwhile applying the principles to your everyday practice anyway because if you practice it now, you'll be brilliant at it by the time you get to part with your £45 registration fee. If nothing else, follow these principles laid down in the Code of Professional Conduct (UKCC, 1992a) and you will be OK.

Each registered nurse, midwife and health visitor shall act, at all times, in such a manner as to:

- safeguard and promote the interests of individual patients and clients;
- serve the interests of society;
- justify public trust and confidence;
- uphold and enhance the good standing and reputation of the profession.

Bit like the scout and girl guide promise isn't it? But nonetheless important.

This chapter also includes a section at the end on whistleblowing. This is a relevant topic that ties into accountability. What you must remember is that this issue *does* apply to you as a student nurse, not just as a qualified nurse.

Some background information

The responsibility for and authority to ensure professional discipline and regulation has been vested in nursing's statutory bodies for many years. However, it was only with the Nurses, Midwives and Health Visitors Act of 1979, which gave rise to the birth of the United Kingdom Central Council for Nursing, Midwifery and Health Visiting (UKCC), that the level at which a registered nurse could perform was formalised, through 'Rule 18' of the act. A mandatory requirement was placed on this new body to establish and improve standards of professional conduct and gave it the authority to do so:

'The powers of the Council shall include that of providing, in such a manner as it sees fit, advice for nurses, midwives and health visitors on standards of professional conduct.'

Section 2(5) Nurses, Midwives and Health Visitors Act 1979

With admirable foresight, the UKCC recognised that some guidance for practitioners would be beneficial. Additionally, it recognised that as professional activity requires a degree of autonomy and independence in practice, personal accountability for these actions would be demanded. Accordingly, in 1984, they introduced the Code of Professional Conduct (which is now in its third edition).

The Code of Professional Conduct was the Council's definitive advice on professional conduct to its practitioners (UKCC, 1992a). It was written to make explicit to practitioners the extent of their accountability and assist them in the exercise of that accountability.

To whom is the nurse accountable?

Dimond (1995) states that the nurse is accountable to the following:

The public – through criminal law.

The employer – through contract law. Being answerable to the employer for breaches in the contract of employment or job description.

The patient – through a duty of care and the common law of negligence, and through civil law.

The profession – through the Code of Professional Conduct and other relevant documents.

ACCOUNTABILITY TO THE PUBLIC

The National Health Service is mainly paid for through public taxation. Therefore, as a nurse, you are accountable to the public to provide a service for which you are employed and to use the available resources appropriately to provide that service.

However, conflicts may arise while trying to achieve this. For example, your employer may have decided that a certain wound dressing will be used in the organisation because it is the cheapest. However, you know that the dressing isn't necessarily the most effective. Therefore, you have to challenge its use, which risks conflict with your employer. But you have a professional responsibility to do this as well as the accountability you have to the public to ensure they get the best value for their money.

Additionally, you are accountable to the public through criminal law. Criminal law is concerned with punishment for an offence, rather than compensation. Therefore, it is unlikely that you will be sued by a patient under criminal law if you injure them inadvertently or negligently (McHale, Fox and Murphy, 1997). If, however, you have deliberately or recklessly caused injury to them they could sue you.

As with any member of the public, if you commit a crime you can be prosecuted for it – it is an offence against society. Accordingly, if you are found guilty of a criminal offence there are systems in place that allow the police or the courts to report you to the Professional Conduct Committee (PCC). Similarly, if you are brought before a PCC due to what could be a criminal offence (such as theft from a patient or unlawful wounding of a patient), then the UKCC can inform the appropriate authorities of this.

> **Example**
>
> Ms K was a 30-year-old Enrolled Nurse General when she was convicted in the Crown Court of a burglary at the home of an elderly patient and sentenced to a term of imprisonment, suspended for two years. The conviction was found to constitute misconduct and her name was removed from the register. (UKCC, 1992b)

ACCOUNTABILITY TO THE EMPLOYER

You are answerable to your employer through your contract of employment. It carries an implicit assumption that you will do what the employer wants by adhering to organisational policies, procedures and guidelines.

You are accountable for the proper and appropriate use of resources. So, for example, eating food designated for patients (even if they don't want it), using hospital stationery for personal use, or undertaking an action not outlined to you through your employer can lead to internal disciplinary action and/or reporting to the UKCC. As a student nurse, you would also have to face the bigwigs who run your course.

And at the end of the day, the doctor is still legally responsible for the patient (NHS, 1992) and the law supports this concept. The doctor diagnoses and prescribes, the nurse carries out his orders (Hayward, 1999), unless she suspects negligence or criminal intent (such as euthanasia) when she would have to refuse to follow orders and make her concerns known.

Scope of professional practice

Although historically and legally doctors have the overall responsibility for the patient, they have 'allowed' nurses to do certain tasks through the process of delegation. They had to be authorised by the employer, training given, competence assessed and a certificate issued. This led, in many instances, to nurses collecting certificates for different tasks within their organisation and, indeed, if they moved to another organisation they usually had to undergo another training and assessment for the same task.

In 1992, the UKCC introduced the Scope of Professional Practice (Scope) (UKCC, 1992c). It recognised that nurses had the potential to develop their role to include aspects of care for which they did not necessarily hold certificates. Woodrow (1996) argues that Scope refocused nursing into an autonomous profession able to make decisions for itself and take responsibility for its own actions. Thus, Scope further reinforced the concept of accountability.

Scope, therefore, has allowed nurses, midwives and health visitors to undertake tasks previously the remit of doctors, as long as they are satisfied the enhanced roles are in the best interests of the patient, not detrimental to fundamental nursing care and that the nurse is skilled and competent to do them. Nurses also have to ensure that they maintain their competence (something not required previously) and acknowledge any limitations.

Conscientious objection

There are two specific areas to which, legally, conscientious objection can be raised:

- abortion – The Abortion Act 1967;
- technological procedures to achieve conception and pregnancy – The Human Fertilisation and Embryo Act 1990.

Common sense would suggest that anyone who has a conscientious objection to these areas would choose not to work in them. This is not so easy as a student nurse. You need to make any objections clear before you are allocated to clinical areas wherever possible. However, many clinical areas are no longer 'dedicated', so a general surgical ward may admit patients who fall into these categories.

Khan and Robson (1999) also suggest that there are some common law grounds where it may be in the your own interests not to participate:

- criminal acts – you can legally refuse to participate in a treatment or procedure you know is criminal in law, for example the administration of a lethal injection for euthanasia purposes;
- negligent acts – if asked to carry out a procedure you believe is likely to cause the patient harm (a negligent act), for example giving the wrong dose of a drug.

ACCOUNTABILITY TO THE PATIENT

This is arguably the most important area of accountability for the nurse. As an autonomous practitioner you are answerable and responsible for the outcome of your professional action. You have a legal and professional duty to ensure that you care for your patients and that the care was given to a certain standard.

The nurse's duty of care

Traditionally, the legal test of a duty of care is based on the 'neighbour principle', and arose out of a case in which a young woman sued a soft drinks manufacturer after finding a partially decomposed snail in a bottle of ginger beer that she had begun to drink (*Donoghue vs Stevenson*, 1932).

The 'neighbour principle' is based on a statement made by Lord Aitkin during the case:

'You must take reasonable care to avoid acts or omissions which you can reasonably foresee would be likely to injure your neighbour.'

In other words, a person has a duty of care to another if they can see that their actions are reasonably likely to cause harm to another person. So a nurse has a duty of care to her patient by virtue of the nurse/patient relationship that she and the patient enter into. *This applies to you as a student.* If a duty of care is breached in some way, either through act or omission, a civil action for negligence may be brought by the patient.

The standard of care

The court determines what would have been a reasonable action in a particular set of circumstances through the application of the Bolam Test:

'The test is the standard of the ordinary skilled man exercising and professing to have that special skill. A man need not possess the highest expert skill at the risk of being found negligent. It is sufficient if he exercises the ordinary skill of an ordinary competent man exercising that particular art.'

(*Bolam vs Friern Barnet Hospital Management Committee*, 1957)

The Bolam Test arose out of case law relating specifically to doctors, but its principles apply to all healthcare professionals, including nurses. Pennels (1998) states that the principle of competence goes hand in hand with accountability because:

- there is an expectation that on completion of basic training the knowledge gained should enable the nurse to function safely;
- the patient should be able to reasonably rely on the practitioner's position and registration in assuming he or she is competent to care for him or her.

This principle applies to all qualified *and student* nurses, regardless of grade or level of experience. In law, being inexperienced is no defence to an action being brought and learners or trainees are judged at the same standard as a more experienced colleague. This was demonstrated in *Nettleship vs Weston* (1971) where it was held that a learner driver must meet the standard of care of a qualified driver, even that of his instructor.

If, however, you seek advice from a more senior or experienced person (which of course you have a responsibility to do if you are unsure of something), then the more senior is accountable. The test case for this principle was that of *Wilsher vs Essex Area Health Authority*. A Senior House Officer inserted an umbilical arterial catheter into a vein instead of an artery, thus giving false oxygen saturation readings. He asked his registrar to check the catheter position. The registrar replaced it, but again into a vein. The baby received too much oxygen and as a result got retrolental fibroplasia. The judge stated that the SHO was not negligent as he was entitled to have his work checked by a senior.

In the course of your practice, there will be issues that arise where you must be aware of your accountability. These include consent and confidentiality.

Consent

The qualified nurse is accountable for ensuring that the patient has given consent for any treatment he or she is giving. Much of the nursing care undertaken is done with implied consent, for example, a patient will roll up his sleeve if you approach with a sphygmomanometer, or open his mouth to have his temperature taken.

It is, however, worthwhile remembering that under civil and criminal law, treating without consent can lead to charges of assault, where the patient is 'in fear' of physical contact without his or her consent, or battery, where the patient is actually touched or treated without permission (Pennels, 1998).

Consent, even implied consent, should only be obtained after you have given the patient adequate information in order for him or her to make a meaningful decision (UKCC, 1996).

The information given to the patient prior to obtaining consent should:

- conform with that which a responsible body of similar professionals in the same speciality would give the patient;
- inform the patient about the nature of the procedure;

- inform the patient of the 'material risks' of the procedure, that is those risks to which a reasonable patient would attach some significance;
- be dictated by circumstance;
- be given without undue influence or duress.

Competent adults can refuse consent. However, if they are suspected to be mentally unfit to give it this refusal can be overruled by the court, for example, *Re T* (1992), where a pregnant Jehovah's Witness refused blood transfusion after going into premature labour and thus needed a caesarean section. Her refusal was overturned by the court in order to protect the baby and the mother.

No person can give consent for another (adult) person and relatives cannot legally give consent for another person except in cases of emergency or mental incompetence. However, this will require a court order.

Similarly, you cannot withhold information from the patient unless the doctor deems it to be detrimental to his or her well-being. Therefore, relatives cannot ask you 'not to tell mum she has cancer'.

For children, the UKCC (1996) advises that as consent of patients under 16 is complex, you should follow local protocols and legislation that affects their treatment. The same should apply to those who are mentally incapacitated and those sectioned under the Mental Health Acts.

Confidentiality

The Code requires you to:

'Protect all confidential information concerning patients obtained in the course of professional practice and make disclosures only with consent where required, by the order of a court or where you can justify disclosure in the wider public interest.' (UKCC, 1992a)

This ties naturally in with the exceptions to the duty of confidentiality:

- by consent;
- by law;
- in the public interest;
- required by the police.

Consent

This may be implied or express. Implied usually refers to the fact that information regarding the patient can be passed between the professionals caring for them. But the patient should be aware that this will happen. This sharing of information should only happen on a 'need to know' basis. Therefore, non-healthcare professionals, such as visiting clergy, have no right to read patients' notes without their consent. Express consent may be obtained in response to circumstances such as telling a relative or friend or the media about the patient's condition.

Law

You have to disclose or withhold information according to certain statutes or specific court orders. These are:

Statutory to disclose information

>Abortion Act 1992
>
>Misuse of Drugs Act 1971
>
>Public Health Act 1984
>
>Prevention of Terrorism Act 1988
>
>Road Traffic Act 1972

Statutory to withhold information

>NHS Venereal Diseases Act 1974
>
>Human Fertilisation and Embryo Act 1990

Court orders

Usually in a civil claim for negligence. The court can order either or both parties to disclose any relevant information or documentation.

Public interest

The UKCC (1996) defines public interest to be 'the interests of an individual, or group of individuals, or of a society as a whole and would cover matters such as serious crime, child abuse, drug trafficking or other activities which could place others at serious risk.'

Whatever the situation you are in, you must be able to justify giving or withholding information. And, as always, it must be documented.

Police

The police can gain access to information under procedures laid down in Schedule 1 of the Police and Criminal Evidence Act 1984.

ACCOUNTABILITY TO THE PROFESSION

You have to act in a professional way whether currently engaged in practice or not and whether on or off duty. So any registered nurse who, for example, decides to take part in a television programme about his or her antics on holiday, or is drunk and disorderly while in uniform, could be seen to be breaking the Code.

You are accountable for keeping yourself up to date in order to ensure that you are a competent practitioner and because you will be passing knowledge on to your peers and subordinates. Additionally, if you do not keep up to date, you will be accountable if a case of negligence is brought against you. In the case of *Hepworth vs Kerr* (1995), it was found that the defendant had failed to keep up to date with a particular procedure and so he was found negligent. However, it is acknowledged that one can't possibly read every text as soon as it is published. The guiding principle must be that you must be up to date with regard to your area of practice and be aware of developments in other areas that may affect your practice.

Clinical supervision

This helps nurses develop skills and knowledge through reflection, support and guidance. However, the supervisor and the supervisee both have accountability and responsibilities within this process.

Supervisors have a professional and contractual duty to report any information given within the supervision session that may constitute a danger to patients (Dimond, 1998).

Although the principle of supervision is that the supervisor helps the supervisee explore issues and alternatives, the supervisor must also be aware of the advice given. It must not be negligent.

If the supervisee is seen to be a danger to the patient and the supervisor does not take any action, he or she will be held accountable if the patient is harmed. If the supervisee feels that the supervisor is giving poor or negligent advice, he or she is accountable for letting someone in authority know. This is in order to protect other colleagues that the person may be supervising and, indirectly, to protect the patient.

Dimond (1998) sums up the accountability issues in supervision thus:

- During supervision, any information disclosing danger to a patient must be followed up.
- Principles of law regarding liability should be taken into account where clinical supervision is practised.
- The supervisee has the same duties in terms of accountability as the supervisor.
- Confidential information may be passed on during clinical supervision and this should be made clear to the patient.
- Clinical supervision records may have to be produced under subpoena.

The principles outlined above could equally apply to the mentorship/preceptorship relationship, so you should be aware of them.

Conclusion

Accountability could be compared to pregnancy – you can't be slightly pregnant and you can't be slightly accountable. The concept of accountability in nursing has been in place for many years. That said, there are still many nurses who are unaware of their accountability or confused by the concept as it applies to them. It is imperative, therefore, that the Code and other UKCC documents are studied and applied to practice.

Unfortunately, the principles contained in the Code are not always clear cut and application may be difficult. However, the nurse must be aware of all aspects of accountability and to whom he or she is accountable, and act accordingly. Ultimately, no matter how many people tell you that they will back you if you 'do X, just this once', once you have done it and it goes wrong, you are the accountable one and the others will have disappeared into the ether. It is better not to have a job but still be on the register than to have no job and no career.

WHISTLEBLOWING

Whistleblowing may be defined as the public disclosure, by a person working within an organisation, of acts, omissions, practices or policies perceived as morally wrong by that person and is a disclosure regarded as wrongful by the authorities of that organisation. For example, a nurse believes that a certain nursing practice is unsafe and reports this to his or her manager. The manager does not act on the report so the nurse takes it higher, and then to the professional body. This body also does not act to the satisfaction of the nurse so he or she then decides to take the report to the union, and it reaches the media. The employer dismisses the nurse for gross misconduct in breaching confidentiality. A legal dispute follows.

Whistleblowing often raises controversy between the employee and the employer about the rightness of the perception of wrongdoing and the justifiability of 'going public'; the nature and scope of corporate, managerial, professional and employee responsibility; the conflicting claims of confidentiality and freedom of speech and of loyalty and honesty; and the openness and accountability of organisations.

The employee may decide to blow the whistle on any matter of moral concern in the workplace that is of general public interest. One may group the majority in terms of:

- danger or detriment to the workforce and/or the public, for example serious infection out of control, shortage or misallocation of patient resources;
- threats to professional integrity and autonomy, for example managerial overriding of professional judgement, research fraud, negligent treatment of clients;
- unfairness or injustice in the workplace, for example sex, race or disability discrimination.

It is useful to distinguish between three foundations, which may overlap:

- Morality – answering to one's conscience in respect of concern for others.
- Professional ethics – answering to one's profession and professional rules.
- The law – answering to the legal and regulatory requirements.

A justifiable disclosure is arguably one which:

- does more good than harm;
- serves some purpose in correcting or preventing the wrongdoing concerned;
- is made in a responsible manner;
- follows on from the exhaustion of internal channels of complaint and redress.

Potential whistleblowers are also well advised to make their disclosure in a responsible manner, if only for the reason that those who object may be inclined to make an issue of the manner, thereby drawing attention away from examining the matter which is being disclosed. This is one aspect of 'shooting the messenger'. Also, someone who is clearly irresponsible in handling a matter is usually less likely to be listened to and believed than someone who handles it with great care.

Responsible disclosure might include:

- making sure one has one's facts right;
- refraining from exaggeration and distortion;
- consulting colleagues;
- avoiding hurt to innocent parties;
- putting aside any inclination to personalise or act vindictively;
- choosing the proper time;
- disclosing to the most appropriate party (someone who is also responsible).

The other side of the coin is that professional nurses have a moral duty to enlighten their managers about the importance of listening to their concerns in a non-defensive and helpful manner. Managers need to ask themselves: what are the conditions under which it is morally, professionally and legally right to *prevent* public disclosure of organisational information? Gagging of staff is unethical. If ignored, staff concerns that may lead to whistleblowing may be treated under certain guiding ethical principles of management (including nurse management)

These might include:

- To consider the concern impartially and establish whether it is true, wholly or in part.
- Not to penalise the conscientious employee for raising a concern even if it is false or misguided.
- To act on a presumption in favour of genuineness on the part of the employee. Even if malice or ulterior motive should emerge, the truth of the whistleblower's claims remains paramount.
- To create positive channels for the expression of concern, such as participatory meetings, exit interviews, rewards for employee vigilance, periodical ethical audits and open door management.
- A readiness to explain and justify to all stakeholders, in a consensus-building spirit, their decisions and actions, for example regarding resource allocation.

In the UK the Public Interest Disclosure Act became law in early 1999. Many believe that whistleblowers are now protected and that victimising employers will be penalised. However, the law is a very weak one because it places the burden of proof on the whistleblower. It is not at all like the anti-discrimination legislation that prevents victimisation on grounds of race, sex and disability. The act only really covers whistleblowing on illegal acts and omissions, and the whistleblower is not protected if he or she commits an offence by whistleblowing, such as legal breach of confidentiality. Under the act the whistleblower would have to show that he or she acted in good faith, that it is reasonable to make the disclosure, that he or she reasonably believed he or she would have been victimised if the concern had been left with the employer, and so on. It would be wise to check the effectiveness of the act with a lawyer before you blow the whistle.

In the last analysis no one can tell you whether you should or should not blow the whistle. It is ultimately a matter of conscience. But there are obligations, differing perceptions and risks and you have to be well informed and well supported.

Support

Support and advice is available from:

Freedom to Care, PO Box 125, West Molesey, Surrey, KT8 1YE
Tel/fax: 020 8224 1022.

References

Bolam vs Friern Barnet Hospital Management Committee (1957), ALL ER 118.

Dimond, B. (1995) *Legal aspects of nursing.* 2nd edition. London: Prentice Hall.

Dimond, B. (1998) Legal aspects of clinical supervision 2: professional accountability. *British Journal of Nursing*; 7: 8, 487–489.

Donoghue vs Stevenson (1932), AC 562.

Hayward, M. (1999) Tug of War. *Nursing Times*; 95: 29, 28–29.

Khan, M., Robson, M. (1999) *A Matter of Conscience.* In: Heywood-Jones, I. (ed.) The UKCC Code of Conduct: a critical guide. London: NT Books.

McHale, J., Fox, M., Murphy, J (1997) *Health care law texts, cases and materials.* London: Sweet and Maxwell.

Nettleship vs Weston (1971), 3 ALL ER 581.

National Health Service (General Medical Services) Regulations SI (1992) *1992/636 Schedule 2: Terms of Service for Doctors (regulations 3 [2]).* London: Department of Health.

Nurses, Midwives and Health Visitors Act 1979. London: HMSO.

Pennels, C. (1997) Nursing and the Law 6: Clinical responsibility. *Professional Nurse*; 13: 3, 162–164.

Pennels, C. (1998) *Nursing and the Law.* London: Professional Nurse Emap Healthcare Ltd.

Re T (1992) Court of Appeal, 3 Med LR 306; 4 ALL ER 649.

UKCC (1992a) *Code of Professional Conduct.* London: UKCC.

UKCC (1992b) *Professional Conduct – Occasional Report on Selected Cases 1 April 1991 to 31 March 1992.* London: UKCC.

UKCC (1992c) *The Scope of Professional Practice.* London: UKCC.

UKCC (1996) *Guidelines for Professional Practice.* London: UKCC.

Woodrow, P. (1996) Professional Practice: the impact of the UKCC practice principles. *Nursing Standard*; 10: 49, 39–41.

Further reading

Heywood-Jones, I. (ed.) (1999) *The UKCC Code of Conduct: a critical guide*. London: NT Books.

Hunt, G. (ed.) (1995) *Whistleblowing in the Health Services*. London: Arnold.

Hunt, G. (ed.) (1998) *Whistleblowing in the Social Services*. London: Arnold.

Khan, M., Robson, M. (1997) *Medical Negligence*. London: Cavendish Publishing Ltd.

Montgomery, J. (1997) *Healthcare Law*. Oxford: Oxford University Press.

Pennels, C. (1998) *Nursing and the Law*. London: Professional Nurse Emap Healthcare Ltd.

Pyne, R.H. (1981) *Professional Discipline in Nursing, Midwifery and Health Visiting*. 2nd Edition. Oxford: Blackwell Scientific Publications.

Tingle, J., Cribb, A. (eds.) (1990) *Nursing Law and Ethics*. Oxford: Blackwell Science.

Young, A.P. (1993) *Legal problems in practice*. London: Chapman Hall.

Young, A.P. (1994) *Law and professional conduct in nursing*. London: Scutari Press.

14 Desperately Seeking Susan – useful contacts

Martin Vousden

Amalgamated School Nurses' Association

60 Shakespeare Crescent, Newport, Gwent NP9 3JE

Professional organisation of school nurses.

Tel: 01633 660897

Association for Continence Advice

ACA

Winchester House, Kennington Park, Cranmer Road, The Oval, London SW9 6EJ

Organisation for all professionals involved in continence care.

Tel: 020 7820 8113

Association for Family Therapy

AFT

c/o Chris Frederick, 12 Mabledon Close, Heald Green, Cheadle, Cheshire SK8 3DB

Open to all professionals.

Tel: 0161 493 9012

Association for Nurse Prescribing

Greater London House, Hampstead Road, London, NW1 7EJ

Independent association to promote nurse prescribing to the professions and others, encourage networking between members and research changes to the nurse prescribers' formulary.

Tel: 020 7874 0350

Association of British Paediatric Nurses

ABPN

c/o Christine Hall, 1 Harley Street, London W1N 1DA

Promoting and furthering the work of paediatric nurses.

Tel: 020 7637 1828 x4417

Association of Nurses in Substance Abuse

ANSA

Carmel Clancy, St George's Hospital, London (Dept of Drug Misuse).

Tel: 020 8725 2585

Association of Nursing Religious

ANR

c/o Sister Catherine Lehane, Sacred Heart of Jesus and Mary Order, Pield Heath House School, Pield Heath Road, Uxbridge, Middlesex UB8 3NW

Member organisation which offers spiritual and professional renewal for Religious in the nursing and caring professions.

Tel: 01895 233092

Association of Occupational Health Nurse Practitioners (UK)

Victoria House, Desborough Street, High Wyecombe, Bucks HP11 2NF

Tel: 01494 601083

Student survival guide

Association of Respiratory Nurse Specialists

ARNS

The Turner Agency, 27 Sturges Road, Wokingham, Berks RG40 2HG

Publishes quarterly supplement in *Nursing Times*.

Tel: 01189 892202

Association of Workers for Children with Emotional and Behavioural Difficulties

AWCEBD

c/o Sue Panter, 20 Carlton Street, Kettering, Northants NN16 8EB

Tel: 01536 513059

Audit Commission

1 Vincent Square, London SW1P 2PN

Appoints auditors to all health authorities and trusts whose job it is to monitor efficiency and cost-effectiveness.

Tel: 020 7828 1212

Benefits Agency

Chief Executive's Office, Room 4CO6, Quarry House, Quarry Hill, Leeds LS2 7UA

Tel: 0113 232 4000

British Association for Immediate Care

BASICS

7 Black Horse Lane, Ipswich IP1 2EF

Tel: 01473 218407

British Association for the Study and Prevention of Child Abuse and Neglect

BASPCAN

10 Priory Street, York YO1 1EZ

A network for professionals.

Tel: 01904 613605

British Association of Critical Care Nurses

BACCN

c/o Greycoat Publishing, 1 Harley Street, London W1N 1DA

Tel: 020 7637 1828 x4417

British Association of Neuroscience Nurses

c/o Anne Murdoch, 1 Parkhall Road, Antrim, Northern Ireland BT41 1BU

Formerly 'British Society of Neurological and Neurosurgical Nurses'. Publishes a twice yearly journal for members.

Tel: 01849 461203

British Association of Parenteral and Enteral Nutrition

BAPEN

Department of Gastroenterology and Nutrition, Central Middlesex NHS Trust, Acton Lane, Park Royal, London NW10 7NS

Tel: 020 8453 2777

Student survival guide

British Association of Urological Nurses

BAUN

c/o Mary Kirkham, Department of Urology, Ward 45, Countess of Chester Hospital, Liverpool Road, Chester CH2 1UL

Tel: 01244 365000 (bleep 2690)

British College of Naturopathy and Osteopathy

Lief House, 3 Sumpter Close, 120–122 Finchley Road, London NW3 5HR

Tel: 020 7435 6464

British Computer Society Nursing Specialist Group

BDNG

PO Box 12, Hadfield, Glossop SK13 2FB

Tel: 01457 865225

British Dermatalogical Nursing Group

BDNG

19 Fitroy Square, London W1P 5HQ

Professional interest group of nurses working or interested in dermatology.

Tel: 020 7383 0266

British Society of Neurological and Neurosurgical Nurses

See 'British Association of Neuroscience Nurses'.

Child Benefit Centre

Newcastle upon Tyne, NE88 1BR

Tel: 0541 555501

Clinical Standards Advisory Group

Room 19, Wellington House, 133–135 Waterloo Road, London SE1 8UG

Established under the 1991 NHS and Community Care Act to advise government of clinical standards, and the quality of access which the public has to health services.

Tel: 020 7972 4918

Commission for Racial Equality

Elliot House, 10–12 Allington Street, London SW1E 5EH

Produces codes of practice and leaflets relevant to NHS employment.

Tel: 020 7828 7022

Committee on Safety of Medicines

Market Towers, 1 Nine Elms Lane, London SW8 5NQ

Established under the Medicines Act 1968 and advises the government regarding safety, quality and efficacy of any substance to which the Medicines Act is applicable.

Tel: 020 7273 0451

Council for Professions Supplementary to Medicine

Park House, 184 Kennington Park Road, London SE11 4BU

Responsible for monitoring standards of education and practice in arts therapy, chiropody, dietetics, medical laboratory services, occupational therapy, orthoptics, physiotherapy, prosthetic/orthotics, and radiography, via professional boards.

Tel: 020 7582 0866

Department of Health

DoH

Richmond House, 79 Whitehall, London, SW1A 2NS

Government health ministry, where the secretary of state for health has his/her office, supported by a minister of state and a number of junior ministers. Also houses the chief nursing and medical officers.

Tel: 020 7210 3000

Department of Health and Social Services (Northern Ireland)

DHSS (NI)

Donaldson House, Newtonards Road, Belfast BT4 3SF

Government department which, in the province, fulfils the function which the departments of health and of social services carry out in England and Wales.

Tel: 028 9052 0500

Department of Social Security

The Adelphi, 1–11 John Adam Street, London WC2N 6HT

Government department responsible for social security matters, including benefits payments.

Tel: 020 7962 8000

Disability Benefits Unit

Warbreck House, Warbreck Hill Road, Blackpool, Lancashire FY2 0YE

Handles all disability living allowance and attendance allowance claims.

Tel: 0345 123456

Employment Service, Disability Services Division

Rockingham House, 123 West Street, Sheffield S1 4ER

Tel: 0114 275 6997

English National Board for Nursing, Midwifery and Health Visiting

ENB

Victory House, 170 Tottenham Court Road, London W1P 0HA

While the UKCC defines the overall standards of nurse education, it is the national boards that ensure these standards are met, by developing, improving and monitoring education courses (both pre- and post-registration). Main responsibility is to provide practitioners with good quality and cost-effective education. Soon to be merged with the UKCC into a single stautory body.

Tel: 020 7383 4031

Environmental Health Departments

See your local telephone directory.

European Network of Occupational Health Nursing

EUROHNET

EUROHNET Secretariat, Oak Ridge, Hook Heath Road, Woking, Surrey GU22 0LF

A peer group network of occupational health nursing teachers and other OH professionals concerned with the development of nurses in occupational health practice.

Tel: 01483 755331

European Oncology Nursing Society

No address available.

Tel: Rira Cautley 00 353 1 282 7255

European Wound Management Association

PO Box 864, London SE1 8TT

Membership open to anyone interested in wound care. Organises conferences, provides money for wound care research and also for travel and education in connection with wound care (excluding conferences abroad).

Tel: 020 7872 3496

Federation of Independent Nursing Agencies

c/o 84 Alma Road, Clifton, Bristol BS8 2DJ

Tel: 01244 315 426

e-mail: fina-facilitator.direct@virgin.net

Useful resource for nursing agencies, agency nursing and PREP

Federation of Mental Health Nursing Organisations

c/o Debbie Murdock, 96 Mickelburgh Avenue, Wells Road, Nottingham NG3 3EL

Tel: 01623 785050 x3418

Forensic Psychiatric Nurses' Association

FPNA

c/o The Raeside Clinic, Birmingham Great Park, Bristol Road South, Birmingham B45 9BE

For mental health nurses working in forensic settings, such as regional secure units and special hospitals.

Tel: 0121 453 6161

Foundation of Nursing Studies

146 Buckingham Palace Road, London SW1W 9TR

Charitable, non-profit making organisation that attempts to bridge the gap between nursing research and practice by disseminating research findings. Any nurse or nursing student can have their name added to the foundation's database and most information is sent out with no charge.

Tel: 020 7824 8182

Desperately Seeking Susan – *useful contacts*

Freedom to Care

PO Box 125, West Molesey, Surrey KT8 1YE

Pressure group established by Graham Pink and Geoff Hunt to support whistleblowers – those who suffer as a result of reporting bad practice – in both health and social services.

Tel: 020 8224 1022

Genito-Urinary Nurses' Association

GUNA

c/o Jeffries Wing, St Mary's Hospital, Praed Street, London, W2 1NY

For nurses interested or involved in genito-urinary or sexually transmitted disease.

Tel: 020 7886 1524

Government Bookshops

For HMSO and other official publications.

Guild of Health (The Church's Ministry of Healing)

Edward Wilson House, 26 Queen Anne Street, London W1M 9LB

Bringing together those who tend the sick through Christianity.

Tel: 020 7580 2492

Health and Safety Commission

Rose Court, 2 Southwark Bridge, London SE1 9HS

Responsible for ensuring the health and safety of people at work, to protect the public against health risks arising from work, and to control the use and storage of explosives. May delegate any of its functions to the Health and Safety Executive.

Tel: 020 7717 6000

Student survival guide

Health and Safety Executive

Rose Court, 2 Southwark Bridge Road, London SE1 9HS

A non departmental public body that sets standards and monitors the implementation of health and safety leglislation in the workplace, particularly in the NHS.

Tel: 020 7717 6000

Health Education Authority

HEA

Trevelyan House, 30 Great Peter Street, London SW1P 2HW

Funded as a special health authority, largely by the Department of Health, to advise on health promotion, undertake research, maintain a knowledge base and work with professionals.

Tel: 020 7222 5300

Health Education Board for Scotland

Woodburn House, Canaan Lane, Edinburgh EH10 4SG

Government body fulfilling the same role as the Health Education Authority in England and Wales.

Tel: 0131 536 5500

Health Information Service

Room 3E58, Quarry House, Quarry Hill, Leeds LS2 7UE

A freephone number (0800) which the public can call for local details about, for example, waiting times for operations and NHS appointments in their area. May eventually be subsumed into 'NHS Direct'.

Tel: 0113 254 6104

Helpline: 0800 665544

Health Promotion Authority for Wales

Ffynnon-las, Ty Glas Avenue, Llanishen, Cardiff CF4 5DZ

Established to hold responsibility for health education and promotion in Wales.

Tel: 029 2075 2222

Health Service Commission

11th Floor, Millbank Tower, Millbank, London, SW1P 4QP

Also known as office of the health service ombudsman. Investigates complaints from health service patients and publishes an annual report of their investigations.

Tel: 020 7217 4051

Health Service Commission for Scotland

1st Floor, 28 Thistle Street, Edinburgh, EH2 1EN

As above.

Tel: 0131 225 7465

Health Service Commission for Wales

Floor 5, Capital Tower, Greyfriars Road, Cardiff, CF1 3AG

As above.

Tel: 029 2039 4621

Holistic Nurses' Association

6 Cornwall Avenue, Rowanfield, Cheltenham, Gloucestershire GL51 8AY

Mutual interest group of nurses committed to, or interested in, holistic care and complementary medicine.

Tel: 020 8650 7510

Human Fertilisation and Embryology Authority

Paxton House, 30 Artillery Lane, London E1 7LS

Set up under the Human Fertilisation and Embryology Act 1990, and is mainly concerned with regulating the storage, research and treatment of human sperm, eggs and embryos.

Tel: 020 7377 5077

Infection Control Nurses' Association

ICNA

c/o Fitwise, Drumcross Hall, Bathgate, Edinburgh EH48 4JT

Publishes bi-monthly supplement in *Nursing Times*.

Tel: 01506 811077

Institute of Allergy Therapists

Llangwyryfon, Aberystwyth, Dyfed SY23 4EY

Professional support organisation that also looks to disseminate best practice.

Tel: 01974 241376

International Council of Nurses

ICN

3 Place Jean Marteau, CH–1201 Geneva, Switzerland

International federation of national nurse representative bodies, which works to spread information about good nursing practice throughout the world.

Tel: 00 41 22 9080100

International Society of Nurses in Cancer Care

c/o Emap Healthcare, Greater London House, Hampstead Road, London NW1 7EJ

Tel: 020 7874 0289

Invalid Care Allowance Unit

Palatine House, Lancaster Road, Preston Lancashire PR1 1NS

Deals with all invalid care allowance claims.

Tel: 01253 856123

Irish Nurses' Organisation (and National Council of Nurses of Ireland)

INO

11 Fitzwilliam Place, Dublin 2, Eire

Representing the views of nurses in Ireland.

Tel: 00 353 1 676 0137

Learning Disabilities Coalition

c/o Brian McGuinness (at Mencap).

Forum of interested organisations, not open to individual members.

Tel: 020 7696 5566

Mental Handicap Nurses' Association

See 'Learning Disabilities Coalition'.

Mental Health Act Commission

MHAC

Maid Marian House, 56 Hounds Gate, Nottingham NG1 1BG

Charged with overseeing the implementation of the Mental Health Act 1983, particularly in regard to protecting the rights of, and investigating complaints from, people who are detained under the provisions of the Act.

Tel: 0115 943 7100

Mental Welfare Commission for Scotland

K Floor, Argyle House, 3 Lady Lawson Street, Edinburgh EH3 9SH

Created by the Mental Health (Scotland) Act 1960, the commission is a standing royal commission, independent of the NHS and Scottish Office. Its broad remit is to protect the interests of people who, by virtue of mental illness, are incapable of adequately protecting themselves.

Tel: 0131 222 6111

Ministry of Agriculture, Fisheries and Food

3 Whitehall Place, London SW1A 2HH

Regulates farming and food production. Operates a helpline for general public enquiries about any of the responsibilities of the ministry.

Tel: 020 7238 6000

Helpline: 0645 335577

Morphine Information Service

Napp Laboratories

Free information and advice for nurses administering morphine. Publishes 'Palliative Care Today'.

Tel: 0800 120012 (freephone)

National Association of Health Workers for Travellers

c/o Joanne Davis, Balsall Heath Health Centre, Edward Road, Balsall Heath, Birmingham B12 9LB

Aims to support staff who are trying to improve the health of travellers.

Tel: 0121 446 4858

National Association of Nurses for Contraception and Sexual Health

25 Ledmore Rd, Charlton Kings, Cheltenham GL53 8RA

Formerly 'National Association of Family Planning Nurses'. Publishes *National Association of Family Planning Journal*.

Tel: 01242 257751

National Association of Theatre Nurses

NATN

Daisy Ayris House, 6 Grove Park Court, Harrogate, North Yorks HG1 4DP

Professional interest group which publishes its own journal, holds conferences and generally works to spread good practice and support members.

Tel: 01423 508079

National Blood Authority

Oak House, Reeds Crescent, Watford, Herts WD1 1QH

A special health authority within the NHS responsible for all blood centres in England.

Tel: 01923 486804

National Board for Nursing, Midwifery and Health Visiting for Northern Ireland

NBNI

RAC House, 79 Chichester Street, Belfast BT1 4JE

See 'English National Board…'.

Tel: 028 9023 8152

National Board for Nursing, Midwifery and Health Visiting for Scotland

NBS

22 Queen Street, Edinburgh EH2 1NT

See 'English National Board…'.

Tel: 0131 226 7371

Student survival guide

National Health Service Executive

NHSE

Quarry House, Quarry Hill, Leeds LS2 7UE

An integral part of the DoH, the NHSE is the headquarters of the NHS. It is responsible for the effective management of the NHS and advises ministers on policy.

Tel: 0113 254 5000

National Radiological Protection Board

Chilton, Didcot, Oxon OX11 0RQ

Set up under the Radiological Protection Act 1970 to investigate and report on the best ways to protect people from radiological hazards.

Neonatal Nurses' Association

Room 7, Third Floor, Milton Chambers, 19 Milton Street, Nottingham NG1 3EW

Tel: 0115 941 7224

NHS Health Advisory Service

Sutherland House, 29–37 Brighton Road, Sutton, Surrey SM2 5AN

Reports to government on long-term hospital and community facilities for people who are older or mentally ill.

Tel: 020 8642 6421

Nurseline

1st Floor, 8–10 Crown Hill, Croydon, Surrey CR0 1RZ

Independent advice, information and support service for all nurses and midwives, provided by the RCN.

Tel: 020 8681 4030

Professional and Practice Development Nurses' Forum

For those nurses interested in all aspects of practice development.

Tel: Jane Mallett 020 7352 8171

Professional Association of Nursery Nurses

PANN

2 St James' Court, Friar Gate, Derby DE1 1BT

Professional interest group exchanging ideas and networking among nursery nurses.

Tel: 01332 343029

Royal National Pension Fund for Nurses

RNPFN

Burdett House, 15 Buckingham Street, London WC2N 6ED

Offers pensions, life assurance and other financial services exclusively for members of the caring professions and their spouses.

Tel: 020 7839 6785

Scottish Office (Home and Health Department)

St Andrew's House, Edinburgh EH1 3DE

Equivalent body to the Department of Health in England and Wales. Soon to be replaced, following devolution.

Tel: 0131 556 8400

Social Security and Child Support Commissioners England and Wales

5th Floor, Newspaper House, 8–16 Great New Street, London EC44 4DH.

Operates the same service as the health service commission, but for social security.

Tel: 020 7353 5145

Student survival guide

Social Security and Child Support Commissioners Northern Ireland

Lancashire House, 5 Linenhall Street, Belfast BT2 8AA

See above.

Tel: 028 9033 2344

Social Security and Child Support Commissioners Scotland

23 Melville Street, Edinburgh EH3 7PW

See above.

Tel: 0131 225 2201

Society of Occupational Health Nursing

c/o Carol Bannister, 20 Cavendish Square, London W1M 0AB

For nurses in, and interested in, occupational health.

Tel: 020 7409 3333

United Kingdom Central Council for Nursing, Midwifery and Health Visiting

UKCC

23 Portland Place, London W1N 4JT

Governing body for nursing, midwifery and health visiting in the UK; maintains the register of all those qualified to practise. Primary responsibility is to protect the public through establishing and improving standards of education, maintaining professional standards and investigating misconduct. Soon to be replaced by another body, details of which will be known in 1999.

Tel: 020 7637 7181

United Kingdom Transplant Support Service Authority

Fox Den Road, Stoke Gifford, Bristol BS34 8RR

A special health authority which maintains records of all patients awaiting organ donation in the UK.

Tel: 0117 975 7575

Welsh National Board for Nursing, Midwifery and Health Visiting

WNB

Second Floor, Golate House, 101 St Mary Street, Cardiff CF1 1DX

See 'English National Board...'.

Tel: 029 2026 1400

Welsh Office

Crown Buildings, Cathays Park, Cardiff, CF1 3NQ

Government department responsible for administration of government business in Wales, at the direction of the Welsh secretary of state. The NHS Directorate, which is part of the Welsh Office, sets the policy agenda for the five Welsh health authorities and 30 trusts. (To be replaced by Welsh parliament in 2000, following elections in 1999.)

Tel: 029 2082 5111

Work Injured Nurses' Group

WING

WING, 8–10 Crown Hill, Croydon, Surrey CR0 1RZ

Self-help group run by its members and coordinated by the RCN. Also open to non-RCN members.

Tel: 020 8649 9536

Wound Care Society

PO Box 170, Huntingdon PE18 7PL

Publishes six wound care supplements a year in *Nursing Times*.

Tel: 01480 434401

15 Reality Bites – what to expect once you qualify

Tony Makepeace

If you read *Nursing Times* any week, there are always hundreds of jobs advertised. Trusts up and down the UK are looking for qualified staff.

After qualifying as a nurse you are a special commodity. Both the diploma and degree are difficult and challenging. Few other academic courses involve such a large practical workload. Perhaps fewer still, if any, involve the emotional and stressful demands of caring for other people as nursing does. You will have earned the right to take on the special role that is nursing.

This chapter has been written to tell you first that it is worth it. Although after qualifying nursing remains physically and emotionally tiring, it is still a job that offers rewards that few others can. The pleasure of interacting with other people, being able to be a positive influence for them is something that few other professions can offer in the same way. Second, this chapter will guide you through the qualifying process; the administration, the job application and the interview process. Finally, it looks at what life is like on the other side, the demands of being a newly qualified staff nurse, the inherent pressures and, crucially, how to avoid them.

REGISTRATION

The period between passing the final assessment and starting the first job is busy. Applying for vacancies, moving home, interviews, even end of

Reality Bites – what to expect once you qualify

course parties all have to be crammed in. During this time there is an application form from the UKCC. It would be easy to set it aside and forget about it, but this form needs prioritising. It is only once the UKCC has received your application form and the 'Declaration of Good Character' has been forwarded from your university that you are allowed to practise. The period of time between qualifying and UKCC registration is a strange stage of limbo – you are neither a student nor a nurse. In this time there are restrictions on practice and the pay is often not the same as that of a staff nurse. The sooner the registration document is sent off the better.

WHICH JOB?

There may be hundreds of jobs from which you can choose. But selecting and winning the right one cannot be over emphasised. It should be one that fits into your long-term plans and gives you the best start to your career.

You will have to consider whether to stay at the hospital where you completed your placements or move to another. If you stay it will ease your introduction to the wards as you already know the systems, locations of equipment and paperwork. However, moving to a different hospital will broaden your knowledge by offering new approaches.

There is the consideration of whether it is worthwhile to move to a completely different part of the country or stay where you are. Your home offers support structures you have already developed. Family, friends and colleagues will provide support and comfort to deal with the inevitable stress of a new ward. Alternatively, a new area presents new experiences and opportunities in nursing and the outside world.

There is the question of whether a fresh ward will offer better experience than one where you enjoyed a placement. New wards will offer new experiences. New colleagues will have fewer preconceived ideas about you. On the other hand, your current ward will treat you differently once you become a staff nurse. A ward where you have worked before will offer more security. Bonds that you have developed with staff members will be useful in the stressful periods ahead. The grass might not be greener on other wards.

It is worth deciding whether a general ward would be a good place to start or whether specialising straight away would be wiser in the long term. A general ward will provide wide experience that will always be transferable in the future. Patients and clients in specialist areas have other problems that you will have to deal with. If you specialise too early, opportunities in future posts may be restricted due to insufficient experience. Alternatively a specialist ward will allow you to work in a field that you know you enjoy. You can focus your energies on learning a restricted area and not rush to know everything too soon.

Rotational posts are currently very popular. They provide wide experience and an organised learning programme. They do have weaknesses in that it can be frustrating to become settled in a team and then have to move on.

It is not an easy choice. There is a wide range of opportunities for newly qualified staff nurses. No one can make the decision for you. The best approach is to obtain as much information as possible. Find out further details about vacancies: arrange a visit to the work area, talk to people who work there and look at the brochures available. Speak to newly qualified staff nurses, find out about their experiences and what advice they would give. Talk to friends for their opinion of what they feel you would enjoy. Wait before making the final decision. Attend interviews for a number of posts so that different options are available. Importantly, take time to reflect before making any decisions.

THE APPLICATION FORM

The application form is normally the first impression that employers receive of you (Ryan, 1993). It is an opportunity to create the right impression and win an interview. While there are many nursing posts available, the good ones are highly competitive. It is vital to present the right image.

Some rules of completing application forms are common sense: neatness, accurate spelling and clarity. Double-check the spelling of any words you are unsure about. Practise answering questions on photocopies of application forms to ensure that responses fit into the space provided.

An application form is intended to demonstrate your experience and ability. Analyse the job specification and tailor answers to this. Surprisingly a lot of people do not do this (Ryan 1993). As a student you will not yet have fulfilled all the attributes of a staff nurse. An application form is an opportunity to demonstrate how past experiences and transferable skills prove that you can mature into the role.

THE INTERVIEW

Everybody is nervous before an interview – it is a natural human response. Whether a person is applying to be the boss of the UKCC, or for a first post, he or she will be nervous. The challenge is to control the nerves sufficiently to use them to your own advantage. Interviewers understand the anxiety of interviews; they have been through many themselves. They will want interviewees to be as comfortable as possible so that they can do themselves justice in the interview.

Whichever job is applied for, some attributes are common. For the interview you should be punctual, smartly dressed, polite and friendly. However good your application form, arriving late, not dressing smartly or being rude and unapproachable will ruin your chances. Once in the interview, demonstrating you have an approachable personality will 'carry you on a carpet of goodwill' (Kennedy, 1996). Being pleasant, sincere and open in your responses and body language will help the interviewer to develop a positive impression of you.

When answering questions it is important to remember the person specification on the application form. Answers need to be geared accordingly so that the interviewers can see the candidate that fulfils their criteria. On top of your achievements as a nursing student, they will want to see the potential and ability to develop, and cope with the transition to being qualified.

Although every interview is different, some questions are regularly asked, especially for newly qualified staff nurses. While you cannot prepare the perfect response to all questions, it is useful to have an idea as to how you will answer the more common ones. That way you will not be surprised and your answer will have more clarity.

Common questions include:

- Tell us about yourself.
- Why do you want this post?
- Why did you become a nurse?
- Where do you want to be in a year's time? In five years' time?
- Do you prefer working in a team or on your own?
- What is your greatest strength? Weakness?

Student survival guide

- What experiences do you have of stressful situations?
- What current issues do you think will most affect nursing?
- How do you think the trust should respond to a specific local issue?
- Tell us how you have overcome a problem?
- What strategies do you use to develop your practice?
- How do you cope with stress?

These questions allow you, the interviewee, to show the prospective employers your skills, experiences, priorities and achievements. All the positive characteristics that make you the person the interviewers are looking for.

Occasionally interviewers throw in difficult and nasty questions – questions for which it is impossible to prepare. One friend of mine was asked to name all parts of the 'Code of Conduct'. The purpose of such questions is not necessarily what you answer, but how you cope with the question. Can you think on your feet? Can you deal with the pressure? The solution is to take time, request a second to think and ask questions for further details. This will give you more time to formulate answers.

At the end of most interviews, it is good practice for interviewers to ask interviewees if they have any questions. This is a further opportunity to discuss interests, skills and issues that will demonstrate to interviewers that you are the ideal candidate for the post. It gives you an opportunity to find out further information about the role. Always prepare a couple of questions. Positive questions on areas such as further training, clinical supervision, preceptorship, local issues or developments within the trust are advisable. This will demonstrate you have an interest in your work and the organisation for which you want to work. Issues such as pay, time off and social activities are seen as frivolous.

PRECEPTORSHIP AND 'REALITY SHOCK'

While it is impossible to gauge the satisfaction that comes from qualifying and finally working as a staff nurse, it is a difficult, stressful time. There are problems to overcome: areas of personal weakness; the difference between the high standards taught in college and those in practice due to working conditions; lack of clinical experience; joining a new team and new responsibilities as a team leader (Charnley, 1999). Kramer (1974) described this as 'reality shock' – the phenomenon by which nurses find themselves in a job for which they are trained, only to find they have not been prepared sufficiently.

As a response, nursing's central bodies advocate a period of preceptorship: 'To help practitioners to achieve confidence in the early months of registered practice a period of support, under the guidance of a preceptor, is recognised.' (UKCC, 1994)

Preceptorship can take many forms: highly organised or more fluid; the responsibilities of one mentor or the whole ward; through rotation of wards or on just one. But essentially, when choosing a first post, the level of support available should be one of the biggest factors in the decision. Support through the first few months after qualifying should be a right. It is in any newly qualified staff nurse's self interest to insist on it. It is in the ward's interest to smooth the transition after qualifying to ensure that new members of staff feel comfortable and are working to appropriate standards.

If it is possible, it helps to develop good personal relationships with a preceptor and other senior staff as a trusting relationship provides more support. In the period immediately post qualification, having colleagues to turn to reduces the many pressures (Maben and MacLeod Clark, 1996a). Asking for advice and discussing areas of weakness is often a difficult task. New staff nurses are often not as prepared as they felt they were. It takes a level of trust and confidence to ask other staff for help when addressing areas of need. It is in those times when a good preceptor is vital. Experienced staff provide direction, teaching and support. It is often here that mentors and role models are found.

The support of other colleagues, more experienced 'D' grades and health care assistants, is also invaluable. In the day-to-day work they are often the ones with whom newly qualified staff nurses work closely. They can assist in orienting the new staff member to the ward, in locating equipment, in understanding the roles of different staff and in learning new methods of working. 'D' Grades will have often recently experienced similar challenges. Fellow students who graduated at the same time are also useful as they share the same experiences at the same time. The opportunity to empathise and let off steam is a welcome one. Everybody needs to reduce their stress by releasing their anxieties.

It is known for newly qualified staff nurses to develop 'staff nursitis' – an over inflated sense of their own self-importance. This is discouraging for new colleagues, and will lead to the new starter losing his or her valuable input.

The ability to cope with stress is one of the biggest factors determining the enjoyment and success of the first few months as a qualified nurse. Emotions have traditionally been seen as a weakness in nursing, perhaps because of the Anglo-Saxon hierarchical tradition of nursing. The situation has improved and there is more awareness that nurses are human too (Bond, 1994). It is now more acceptable to need support and colleagues are well aware of the problems after qualifying. They should be willing to assist in supporting newly registered nurses. There are many other ways of coping: methods include exercise, hobbies, spirituality, or even unconventional acts such as using punch bags or smashing plates. Whatever combination of these is used, it is necessary to find ways to deal with stress. The difficult incidents and taxing issues are helpful in a nurse's development. They provide an opportunity for emotional and professional maturation. Even if a stressful event is poorly dealt with, it provides evidence of a need to develop alternative coping strategies.

After first qualifying it is difficult to adjust to the new role. It is always worth remembering that by qualifying you will have earned the right to be a registered nurse, experienced difficult stages of the course and passed the placements and exams. The assessors of all the placements and the lecturers at university have felt that you were capable of being a registered nurse. 'Reality shock' is a complicated stage to go through, but it is achievable.

PROJECT 2000

In the past year the academic content of pre-registration education has hit the headlines again. Newspaper commentators have been deriding 'Project 2000' and calling for a longer content of practical training in pre-registration courses (Payne, 1999). However, the UKCC is currently investigating nurse education and analysing its future development.

When the early students with a diploma qualified, many faced prejudice and resentment from established nurses. This has now largely gone. The early diploma students are now moving up into 'E', 'F' and 'G' grades. All staff nurses are used to working with diploma nurses. The importance of education is now more accepted than before. There are still many different opinions about pre-registration education (Munro, 1999; Butler, 1999), but new staff nurses no longer face a blanket of prejudice.

EDUCATION

Learning does not stop after qualifying; in fact it accelerates. The period of settling in to the new role requires rapid knowledge acquisition. This is a vital part of any preceptorship programme. The preceptor and other staff should be open to questions, they should encourage new staff to develop their expertise and assist with clinical skills. But ultimately it is the newly qualified staff nurse's responsibility to develop his or her knowledge. Lifelong learning is now a prerequisite for continuing practice with PREP requirements. Nurses are directly accountable for their own learning. It is important to access educational opportunities, courses at your own trust and outside and research published in the professional journals that has been experienced by specialist staff. This is invaluable for developing practice and experience.

Reflection is a key to the development process (Atkins and Murphy, 1993). Everybody reflects on their life, but to be constructive at work it needs to be 'intentional and purposeful' (Andrews, 1996). Some people use reflective diaries to record their experiences; others discuss incidents and events with a colleague. Colleagues can offer their experience and peers can provide support to help identify feelings, alternative strategies and outcomes of an event. I used to take home lists of issues I felt weak on, medications with which I was not familiar and diseases I did not understand. Initially the lists were huge, but gradually as my experience and knowledge increased, the lists shrank. Whatever level of experience I reach, I will always need to address where I need to develop my knowledge and the lists will continue.

MONEY

One of the joys of qualifying is the thought of the money. The student years are a period of building up debt, denial and reliance on other people, and for most students they are. Everybody knows someone who manages to make a profit. Student funding is insufficient, be it for diplomas or degrees. The future with a good salary is something to look forward to in the dark days when there is only one tin of baked beans left until pay day.

Unfortunately, the salary of a staff nurse is never sufficient. After three years on a pittance one would imagine that it is easy to live on a staff nurse's earnings. But it seems that there is never enough money to last to the end of the month. It is often back to those baked beans. This year's pay award left the starting salary at £14,400. When compared to a student bursary this is a very liveable wage – it just needs to be treated with caution. It would be easy to buy that new car, go for the holiday in Marbella instead of Morecambe or move to a nicer part of town. This will hit the bank balance very hard and lock you into some serious debt. On graduation, banks become very friendly – loans, special accounts and mortgages are readily offered. But these all need repaying. The quality of junk mail improves – somehow companies realise that you have a larger disposable income.

The demands on your finances automatically increase. Student discounts no longer apply, whether they were at the local clothes shop or the nightclub. Moving out of the nurses' home means moving into rented accommodation or your own home. The rent/repayments will be a lot larger. When the bills and community charge start coming through it is even worse.

On top of all that there is tax. Students who have worked full time before will not be surprised at the amount of tax taken. The combination of National Insurance and income tax appears huge compared to the small amounts taken from part time jobs. The £14,400 is not as large as it appears.

The first month's salary is often smaller than expected. Some trusts pay at healthcare assistant salaries until the UKCC registration arrives. It is only then that the first month(s) shortfall is repaid.

Nevertheless, the larger income does provide more opportunities. It is great to be able to buy better food, pay off debts, purchase items that you have denied yourself through training and move to a nice flat. But it is important to remember that debt is an easy trap to get into, and even harder to escape from.

CONCLUSION

The first few months as a staff nurse are a shock. Being a nurse is a difficult job. It is hard work; not how most people imagine it and there is a lot to learn. But after all the struggle to qualify – the difficult placements, exams, essays, emotional and stressful times of pre-registration education – the stress after qualifying is not surprising. This is why nursing students have to work so hard and why nursing is valued so greatly by society.

Efforts can be made to minimise the stress. Choosing and acquiring the right job for you will help you to feel more comfortable. Learning to trust and rely on new colleagues helps to access the support of experienced staff – individuals who know what you are suffering because they have been there. It is useful to have friends to talk to and methods of relaxing to avoid letting work affect your home life. Most of all be willing to learn. Pre-registration education is only the start. Learning never stops as a nurse. In the first few months as a staff nurse it is very rapid. Then, after a few months it does become easier. Confidence increases and people gain more trust and respect for you. Opportunities increase and you move on to the next stage of your career.

References and further reading

Andrews, M. (1996) Using reflection to develop clinical expertise. *British Journal of Nursing*; 5: 8, 508–513.

Atkins, S, Murphy, K. (1993) Reflection: a review of the literature. *Journal of Advanced Nursing*; 18,1188–1192.

Bond, M. (1994) *Stress and Self Awareness: a Guide for Nurses*. Oxford: Butterworth Heinemann.

Bowles, N. (1995) A critical appraisal of preceptorship. *Nursing Standard*; 9: 45, 25–28.

Butler, N. (1999) Baby out with the bathwater. Letter to the Editor. *Nursing Times*; 95: 4, 18.

Castledine, G. (1996) Is preceptorship the answer to reality shock? *British Journal of Nursing*; 5: 10, 641.

Chaffer, D. (1999) The great education debate. *Nursing Standard*; 13: 22, 22–23.

Charnley, E. (1999) Occupational stress in the newly qualified staff nurse. *Nursing Standard*; 13: 29, 33–36.

Clutterbuck, D. (1994) *Everyone needs a Mentor: Fostering Talent at Work*. 2nd Edition. London: Institute of Personal Development.

Cudmore, J. (1999) Make me welcome in your world. *Nursing Times*; 95: 9, 24.

Eaton, A. (1999) Too clever to care? *Nursing Times*; 95: 4, 14–15.

Ellis, E. (1999) Let's call a halt. *Nursing Times*; 95: 4, 18.

Gardner Huber, D. (1994) What are the sources of stress for nurses? In: McCloskey, J., Grace, H. (eds). *Current Issues in Nursing*. 4th Edition. St Louis, Missouri: Mosby.

George, S. (1999) Back to the future. *Nursing Times*; 95: 1, 62–63.

Gerrish, C. (1990) Fumbling along. *Nursing Times*; 86: 30, 35–37.

Gillan, J. (1999) Bedside manner misses the point. *Nursing Times*; 95: 4, 22.

Kennedy, J. (1996) *Job Interviews for Dummies*. Foster City, California: IPD Books Worldwide.

Kramer, M. (1974) *Reality Shock: Why Nurses Leave Nursing*. St Louis, Missouri: Mosby.

Law, D. (1994) So, why do you want this job? *Nursing Standard*; 8: 46, 52.

Maben, J., MacLeod Clark, J. (1996a) Making the transition from student to staff nurse. *Nursing Times*; 92: 44, 28–31.

Maben, J., MacLeod Clark, J. (1996b) Preceptorship and support for staff: the good and the bad. *Nursing Times*; 92: 51, 35–38.

McHaffie, H. (1992) Coping: an essential element of nursing. *Journal of Advanced Nursing*; 17, 933–940.

Melia, K. (1987) *Learning and Working: the Occupational Socialisation of Nurses*. London: Tavistock Publications.

Morton-Cooper, A., Palmer, A. (1993) *Mentoring and Preceptorship: a Guide to Support Roles in Clinical Practice*. Oxford: Blackwell Scientific Publications.

Munro, R. (1999) Could do better. *Nursing Times*; 95: 1, 60–62.

Payne, D. (1999) The knives are out. *Nursing Times*; 95: 4, 14–15.

Ryan, T. (1993) Job search: the science of success. *Nursing Standard*; 7: 49, 44–45.

Simpson, P. (1999) Educated for better care. *Nursing Times*; 95: 4, 18.

Turner, C. (1998) Qualified to patronise. *Nursing Times*; 94: 40, 68.

United Kingdom Central Council for Nursing, Midwifery and Health Visiting (1998) *Guidelines for Higher Education Institutions on Registration for Newly Qualified Nurses and Midwives*. London: UKCC.

United Kingdom Central Council for Nursing, Midwifery and Health Visiting (1998) *The Future of Professional Practice – the Council's Standards for Education and Practice Following Registration*. London: UKCC.

16 Carry on Nurse
– nursing howlers

Phillip Hufton

Yes, this is a very serious time in your lives, but it can also be one of the happiest. You will get out of the next three years what you put into it. I can tell you from personal experience that you should put the maximum in, and you will get the maximum out. Get involved in everything that goes on around you – educational and professional committees, clubs and societies, social and sporting events... Everything!

Work hard, but be sure to find time to enjoy yourself as well. Don't be one of those resentful types who spends all the time saying 'we never had the time to do anything like that in our training!', and believe me, you will meet them. Just be sure to tell them 'Rubbish', it is what you make it, and it is up to you.

Of all the important ingredients you will need during your training, a good sense of humour is probably one of the most important. Be sure to pack it, along with your other belongings. The ability to laugh in the face of doom and gloom, when all around you is stress and strain, to laugh with others and, above all, to be able to laugh at yourself, will hold you in good stead for the next three or four years, and hopefully long after that. To find humour in adversity will be your strength.

With that in mind, in this chapter I hope to share some gems from the annals of nursing and hospital times past. They have been collated from various sources too numerous to mention, and while the jokes speak for themselves, the care plan quotes are all, as far as we know, quite genuine.

Care plan quotes

'My patient learned to ambulate to the bathroom, bend at the knees and eat himself.'

'The patient stated that he had got a bone stuck in his throat. This was obviously because he had not masturbated his food properly.'

'The patient got out of bed, while the nurses stripped.'

'The man was sometimes violet towards her.'

'The nursing staff will discuss the patients sleeping with the night staff.'

'The nurse will chart the patient's weight on Mondays, wearing daytime clothes without shoes after breakfast.'

'Initially, because of his large moist size, it was a problem fitting his trousers.'

'I arranged his trousers, but his shit was still hanging out.'

'A bed cradle was put in situ, to take the weight off her legs and cause considerable pain.'

'After a while the patient was reduced to walking with two crutches, two walking sticks, and a stick.'

'Some illnesses are inherited, others run in families.'

'Prior to a barium enema the doctor may need a rectal washout.'

'Carrying the heavy object caused him to have a bi-lingual hernia.'

'On commencement of treatment the patient should be taken into the treatment room, put onto a bed, and someone will get familiar with them.'

'The assessment technique used on the ward consists of an objectionable client assessment.'

'The patient was asked to wash his own top half including his genitals at the side of the bed.'

'The patient should prevent periods of standing when in bed.'

'The patient should be given 500ml a day to drink, plus yesterday's output.'

'Death only occurs in fatal cases.'

Student survival guide

'Ensure that the patient can eat himself.'

'Prior to the barium enema, the patient's rectum should be blown up.'

'The four steps for resuscitation are:
1. Take pulse
2. Ring crash team
3. Get them on the floor
4. Resuscitate'

'In an emergency arrest:
1. Lay patient on a firm surface head back. Remove obstructions to the mouth.
2. Put fingers on pulse, bang sternum.
3. One bang on chest, check pulse.
4. One blow in mouth, five on chest.'

'In old age, blood vessels become thin and electric.'

'The nurse herself can prevent cross infection by good standards of hand washing after handling contaminated diet, like bedpans.'

'In her previous life, she experienced no problems.'

'Sister Anna Maria, a Catholic nun, who is currently in between missionary positions.'

'The patient had had twelve children by her doctor.'

'Nursing staff should maintain a safe environment by avoiding contact with patients.'

'Female clients may not like the males being there interfering with them.'

'Put head back, hold nose, and give five good hard blows to the mouth.'

The pyrexial patient should not wear make up if she is expiring.'

'Highly medicated patients are undesirable.'

'After his bath the patient was assisted into his gown with a nurse.'

'Despite his death the patient was progressing well.'

'The blanket was removed and replaced with a nurse.'

'Sexually uninhibited behaviour would be included in the plan of care.'

'Encourage the patient to eat. If he does not, supplement the diet with smacks.'

'Anxiety can cause many symptoms, for example hair standing upright on the patient's neck and shoulders.'

'The nurse will observe the patient's trousers for abnormal swellings.'

'The nurse must bear in mind that people belong to different religions, such as Muslims, Jews, and Genitals.'

'Some patients who have a circumcision get upset, others just laugh it off.'

'The nurse laid him, on the floor.'

'The patient has had problems with vision for days, and the doctor told him that this was as a result of a detached rectum.'

'You can develop confidence by exposing yourself to the patient.'

'On the way to theatre the nurse should re-insure the patient.'

'Weil's disease is carried by rats that are excreted in the urine.'

'The laundry of an infected patient should be double bagged, along with a nurse.'

'He weighed 75 kilograms, which was a satisfactory weight, for his weight.'

'Medication to control moods should be taken by the registered nurse.'

'To explain the future risks to the patient, we should start with a heavy session of alcohol abuse.'

'It is always advantageous to gain inexperience in these matters.'

'The patient had been depressed since I had started nursing her.'

'If only a small branch of the heart is blocked, the region of the heart muscle becomes neurotic.'

Student survival guide

'Reasons for catheterisation:

a) Before or after pregnancy

b) Before or after surgery'

'The patients themselves might start an infection, by being inquisitive, and having a peep under a sterile dressing, and using their fingers, which may have earlier been used for turning the pages of a dirty book.'

'During sleep the body gets to work repairing and maintaining any damaged tissue, and frightening any infection.'

'Hourly observations must be recorded every half hour.'

'Poor appetite and weight loss reduce bodyweight.'

'Tepid sponging can take place by splitting the body in three parts.'

'The nursing officer was appalled by the cleanliness of the ward.'

'Some patients come into hospital to die, which can be a very tense time for them.'

'I calmed her down by calling her names quietly.'

Exam question: From what may men in their fifties suffer?
Answer: The manopause.

Exam question: What is a common treatment to prevent a bleeding nose?
Answer: Circumcision.

Exam question: How should nurses prepare a patient before a pre-med injection?
Answer: They must wash the patient's groin and genial areas.

Exam question: How can parents help when a child wakes in the night, suffering from breathing difficulties?
Answer: Make them inhale a kettle.

Carry on Nurse – nursing howlers

What does it all mean?

Artery – the study of paintings

Bacteria – back door to a cafeteria

Cat scan – Searching for a kitty

Coma – a punctuation mark

Cauterise – made eye contact

D&C – where Washington is

Fibula – a small lie

Genital – not Jewish

Pelvis – cousin of Elvis

Prostate – flat on your back

Seizure – a Roman emperor

Secretion – hiding something

Terminal illness – getting sick at the airport

Tibia – a country in North Africa

Vein – conceited

Postoperative – letter carrier

Pap smear – fatherhood test

Labour pain – work related injury

Recovery room – place to do upholstery

Tumour – more than one

Ten things that consultants never say

- Sorry.
- I've never worn a bow tie, and don't intend to start.
- How about paying us based on the success of the project?
- This whole strategy is based on a paper that I read in *The Lancet*.

Student survival guide

- Actually, the only difference is that we charge more than they do.
- I don't know enough to speak intelligently about that.
- No, I insist, I'll bring the biscuits/cakes next week.
- I can't take the credit; it was all nurse X's doing.
- The problem is you have too much work, and too few nurses.
- Nurses are in a much better position than me to make a judgement on that.

Question: When a consultant dies, why do you bury him 12 feet down?
Answer: Because deep, deep, down, they are all really nice people.

Question: What's black and brown, and looks good on a consultant?
Answer: A rottweiler

Question: How do you get a consultant out of a tree?
Answer: Cut the noose.

Question: What does a consultant use for birth control?
Answer: His personality.

A man died and was taken to his place of eternal torment by the devil. As he passed sulphurous pits and screaming sinners, he saw a man he recognised as a consultant surgeon, cuddling up to a very beautiful woman.

'That's unfair!' he cried. 'I have to roast for all eternity and that consultant gets to spend it with a beautiful woman.' 'Shut up,' barked the devil, jabbing him with a pitchfork. 'Who are you to question that woman's punishment?'

On the wards

The new auxiliary told the staff nurse that one of the patients had had a good result from the suppositories. 'Put it in the bowel book,' she was told. The next person to open the book had a very unpleasant surprise.

Carry on Nurse – nursing howlers

When Project 2000 started, as many will tell you, it caused a great many problems on the wards, for reasons many and varied. Students, formerly part of the workforce, were now only allowed to go onto the wards and watch what was going on.

One such student was looking at the 'Off Duty' and its puzzling layout of letters and abbreviations. Most she could work out: DO = Day Off; SN = Staff Nurse; WR = Ward Round and so on. However, right at the bottom, before her own surname, was the acronym JAFO. She struggled for a solution, Junior Associate, Junior Allocation and so on. In the end she asked a passing auxiliary. 'Oh that's easy,' he said, 'Just Another F***ing Observer!'

Remember, have confidence in yourself and your abilities, and never, ever take life too seriously. Keep smiling, it will all be worth it in the end.

If you have any contributions, jokes, quotes, or care plan howlers, send them to us at the following address. The best ones will be published and will win a year's **FREE** subscription to *Nursing Times*. Send to:

Phillip Hufton
c/o NT Books Special Projects
EMAP Healthcare
Greater London House
Hampstead Road
London NW1 7EJ

Mark your envelope *Student Survival Guide Howlers*.